INSTITUTIONALISM AND SCHIZOPHRENIA

A COMPARATIVE STUDY OF THREE MENTAL HOSPITALS 1960–1968

OTHER BOOKS BY THE AUTHORS

Brown, G. W., Bone, M., Dalison, B. and Wing, J. K. *Schizophrenia and Social Care*. No. 17 in Maudsley Monograph Series. London: Oxford University Press, 1966.

Wing, J. K. (ed.) *Early Childhood Autism*. Oxford: Pergamon Press, 1967.

Wing, J. K., Bennett, D. H. and Denham, J. *The Industrial Rehabilitation of Long-stay Schizophrenic Patients*. Medical Research Council Memo. No. 42. London: HMSO, 1964.

Wing, J. K. and Bransby, R. (eds.) *Psychiatric Case Registers*, Stat. Rep. Series No 8. London: HMSO, 1970.

INSTITUTIONALISM AND SCHIZOPHRENIA

A COMPARATIVE STUDY OF THREE MENTAL HOSPITALS 1960–1968

J. K. WING

Professor of Social Psychiatry, University of London
Director, Medical Research Council Social Psychiatry Unit,
Institute of Psychiatry, London

AND

G. W. BROWN

Reader in Sociology, Bedford College, London

WITH A CHAPTER BY THE
PHYSICIAN SUPERINTENDENTS
OF THE THREE HOSPITALS

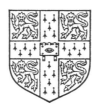

CAMBRIDGE
AT THE UNIVERSITY PRESS
1970

CAMBRIDGE UNIVERSITY PRESS
Cambridge, New York, Melbourne, Madrid, Cape Town, Singapore, São Paulo, Delhi

Cambridge University Press
The Edinburgh Building, Cambridge CB2 8RU, UK

Published in the United States of America by Cambridge University Press, New York

www.cambridge.org
Information on this title: www.cambridge.org/9780521112802

First published 1970
This digitally printed version 2009

A catalogue record for this publication is available from the British Library

Library of Congress Catalogue Card Number: 75–118068

ISBN 978-0-521-07882-5 hardback
ISBN 978-0-521-11280-2 paperback

WITNESS 1
You could only react normally
during your first hours in the camp
When you had been there any length of time
it was no longer possible
You were absorbed into the routine
you were in prison
and you had to make do

Peter Weiss
The Investigation
Canto 2

CONTENTS

TABLES AND FIGURES

The tables and figures are numbered in one sequence, by chapter, and are distinguished in this list by the prefix T or F. Except in Chapters 4 and 6, most of them show the three hospitals separately.

xii *Tables and figures*

T.9.6   Contact with the outside, at Columbia County and
        Mapperley hospitals, 1964   *page* 248
T.9.7   Average time budget at Columbia County and
        Mapperley hospitals, 1964   248
T.9.8   Clinical classification of thirty-eight patients in Columbia
        County and Mapperley hospitals, matched for length of
        stay, 1964   249

PREFACE

This monograph presents the results of part of a programme of research in social psychiatry and is intended to be read in conjunction with other publications from the Social Psychiatry Research Unit (Brown, Bone, Dalison and Wing, 1966; Wing, 1966a; Wing, Bennett and Denham, 1964). The first of these monographs was concerned with schizophrenic patients admitted to the same three hospitals in 1956 and followed up for five years. It is therefore a companion volume to the present one.

Marvin Opler (1967) has complained that the development of a scientific social psychiatry is held up for lack of an Einstein. We feel that the time is hardly ripe for a Copernicus, let alone a Kepler or Galileo, and that our subject has only just reached the threshold of a scientific age. We should be very content if our work were thought merely to have contributed some 'hard and obstinate' facts, after the manner of Tycho Brahe, to a subject where theories are all too easily elaborated but are rarely meant to be tested. Nevertheless, we have worked from a set of interacting social and biological theories which have evolved from a series of investigations into schizophrenia and which we think might prove a useful model for studies of other psychiatric syndromes as well.

We have avoided elaborate statements about statistical significance. Differences have been tested by χ^2 (two-tailed test), by analysis of variance or by non-parametric techniques as appropriate, but none of our conclusions rests on the value of any particular probability. When using parametric statistics we have always looked at the distributions of the variables and made sure, whenever there was any skewing, that the appropriate non-parametric techniques produced a similar degree of significance.

J. K. W.
G. W. B.

ACKNOWLEDGEMENTS

Our first acknowledgement must be to the staff and patients of the three hospitals we studied. We were made very welcome and given every help we asked for. We are particularly indebted to the Principal Nursing Officers Miss Kane (Mapperley), Miss Smith, Mrs Norbury and Mr H. M. Dalton (Netherne), and Miss Clarke and Mr Kniveton (Severalls). Miss Jackson was most helpful in collecting follow-up information on patients who had left Severalls and Mrs Adkin provided data on patients living out at Mapperley. Administrative Officers at all three hospitals (Mr Davies, Mr Hooton and Mr Spalding) were also very co-operative.

Professor Martin Loeb and Dr Peter Weiss made possible the study in Madison, Wisconsin, and Dr Lorna Wing undertook the social measurements there. We are greatly indebted to the Superintendent, Matron and Social Worker of Wyocena County Hospital.

Mrs Margaret Devine, of the MRC Computer Services Centre, has been concerned with the statistical analysis throughout and we are most grateful for her skill and constructive suggestions.

Finally, we should like to acknowledge a very special debt to Dr Barton, Dr Freudenberg and Dr Macmillan. To some extent, in a study of this kind, a physician superintendent must inevitably feel himself, as well as his hospital, under scrutiny, and even under trial. If so, we were never given any hint of it nor was any limitation placed upon our work, and all the suggestions we received were of the utmost practical value in organising our investigation. In return, we hope it is clear from this book that not only was the quality and the dedication of the staff most impressive, but that such problems as were shown up in the study arose from impersonal aspects of social structure and organisation which are, in the first place, difficult to recognise and, in the second place, almost impossible to change without enormous and sometimes unrewarding effort. The potential to take advantage of adequate resources, as they become available to the staff of these hospitals, is already there.

We are very sad to have to record the death of Dr Macmillan on Christmas Day, 1969. He was a great pioneer in his field.

J. K. W. & G. W. B.

1

DISEASE AND THE
SOCIAL ENVIRONMENT

The study reported in this book is concerned entirely with long-stay schizophrenic patients, but the ideas which inspired it, and which it was designed to test, have a much wider relevance. Institutionalism is a sociological concept which can be applied not only to schizophrenia and to mental hospitals, and not only to artificially segregated communities, but to familiar and everyday social events which affect all of us. A study of the relationships between institutionalism and schizophrenia may therefore illuminate problems which are of interest well beyond the confines of medicine, as well as throwing light on matters of contemporary concern or controversy in social psychiatry.

Such wide-ranging interests are a handicap in reviewing the literature because so much in the fields of anthropology, sociology, social psychology, psychology and psychiatry is relevant. We can attempt, in this chapter, only to give a personal (that is, a highly selective) impression of some of the ideas and studies which have influenced us. We are basically interested in the interaction between social and clinical events, so that social psychological and social psychiatric studies will be considered in most detail. The sociology of institutions (particularly of institutions without an ostensibly medical function) must be mainly left aside. This means that methods of structuring the *staff* environment so that patients are treated in an optimally therapeutic way are not discussed in detail. We are mainly concerned with the effect of techniques which could be used by staff to influence patients, rather than with attempts to ensure that these techniques are actually used. That is, we are not primarily interested here in staff organisation or with teaching. Similarly, we shall not deal in detail with many studies which use administrative indices, such as length of stay, to estimate morbidity.

That there is a syndrome of institutionalism, in the narrow sense of personal changes induced by prolonged residence in relatively closed communities, is immediately apparent from numerous novels and memoirs. Thomas Mann, in a long and claustrophobic story about a tuberculosis sanatorium, describes in hypnotic detail the insidious encroachments of institutional life and the gradual disappearance of resistance to its procedures, until the hero (a passive young man who has lost his parents) no longer even considers returning to the world outside. A. E. Ellis in *The Rack* makes the same point: '...it ought to be the most terrible upheaval to come to live in the mountains, to leave everyone and everything one knows and loves, but instead one accepts it, one forgets that one ever lived in any other way and finally one doesn't even seriously think in terms of leaving—it is as though one's past life was something one had once read about in a half-forgotten novel.' Mary McCarthy describes the social and personal reaction when circumstances suddenly change in some appalling way and life can never be the same again. She and her brothers were recovering from the disease which had killed their parents. 'We awoke to reality in the sewing room several weeks later...We became aware, even as we woke from our fevers, that everything, including ourselves, was different. We had shrunk, as it were, and faded, like the flannel pyjamas we wore, which during these few weeks had grown, doubtless from the disinfectant they were washed in, wretchedly thin and shabby. The behaviour of the people around us, abrupt, careless and preoccupied, apprised us without any ceremony of our diminished importance. Our value had paled, and a new image of ourselves—the image, if we had guessed it, of the orphan—was already forming in our minds.'

Albert Camus considers the diverse reactions of the inhabitants of a North African town when the plague suddenly cuts them off from the outside world and they have to face an unknown period of danger and isolation. Primo Levi, in perhaps the most revealing and rewarding of all the personal descriptions of life in a concentration camp, compels his readers to accept that both guards and inmates can react to conditions which permit persecution in ways most people would rather not think about. Authors as far removed from each other as Roy Fuller and George Orwell, Evelyn Waugh and Brendan Behan, have illustrated the changes in attitude that can occur when a vulnerable person is placed into a social environment which requires adherence to an arbitrary and depersonalising routine and limits opportunities to practise normal social roles.

These accounts of the effects of institutions on their inmates are so incomparably superior in literary merit to the descriptive writings of sociologists or psychiatrists that one is tempted to give them greater credit as scientific documents, but that, of course, would be an elementary error. They need no justification apart from their standing as works of art, though they may also serve a reform function: not, perhaps, as immediate as the results of a sensational journalistic exposure but possibly more effective in the long run. Primo Levi's account of a concentration camp, though written in a low key, effectively arouses the emotions so that the reader is determined (for the moment, at least) that such things must never be allowed to happen again. Books which are written specifically to call attention to difficulties in existing institutions have a similar effect.

It is, however, very important to distinguish between the reform of institutions which are obviously pernicious in their effects and the modification of regimes which, ostensibly, have a therapeutic or protective function. To take an example with which we are much concerned in this book: is the commonly described picture of the long-stay schizophrenic patient—shambling, inactive and apathetic—the result of long exposure to an institutional regime or could it occur after the same period of time even if the patient stayed at home? The literary or journalistic method is not well-suited to answering questions of this kind and it could do harm if it provided the incorrect answer. As Lemert pointed out, 'reform movements often create more problems than they solve.' Propaganda, too, can have high literary merit.

Thus the two aims, to prevent inhumane treatment and uphold human dignity on the one hand, and to provide conditions in which handicaps are reduced and assets maximised, on the other, require different approaches and techniques, although in the long run, to achieve the second aim is a means of realising the first. The scientist is not necessarily a reformer and the reformer is usually a poor scientist. Nevertheless, the two aims are not incompatible. In so far as the scientist provides comprehensible and valid information about the effects of institutions, he is laying the foundations for effective reform. We shall not, therefore, be further concerned, in this chapter, with the large and useful literature which is mainly aimed at drawing attention to gross abuses. We are interested in the problems that remain when gross abuses have been corrected or where, happily, they were never present.

INSTITUTIONS AND INMATES

Etzioni (1961) has compared and contrasted various types of complex bureaucratic organisation, which he defines, after Parsons, as 'social units devoted primarily to the attainment of specific goals'. It is useful for those interested in particular communities such as hospitals, to be shown the relevance of others, such as schools, factories, offices, army units, prisons or villages. Etzioni's analysis is most illuminating, but he follows the common practice of American sociologists in classifying mental hospitals as a special variety of coercive institution. It is assumed that 'should the restraints on movement be lifted, hardly any inmate would stay inside'. Since this is manifestly untrue of British mental hospitals, where only 4 per cent of patients are under any kind of legal restriction, it is difficult to use the basic elements of Etzioni's analysis—power, involvement and compliance—according to his specifications. Indeed, the functions of mental hospitals are so varied (Clark, 1956) that the only practicable plan seems to be to single them out one at a time for investigation. It might then appear that, in certain respects, a mental hospital is like a school, in others like a commercial firm, in others like a general hospital, in others like a prison and in yet others like an asylum or retreat.

There is, however, the complication that all British mental hospitals have passed through a 'custodial' period, in which most patients were under legal order, and a major aim—though not the sole aim—was to ensure quiet behaviour and a minimum of escapes. Large changes have taken place since then, but the long-stay patients remain from the old days.

Goffman (1961) has drawn attention to the way in which such 'old-fashioned' mental hospitals resemble other segregated communities in which inmates are isolated from general social life. Such 'total institutions' tend to develop practices which bear a remarkable similarity to each other. The staff and inmates have fundamentally different points of view, and may come to perceive each other in narrow, hostile stereotypes. There is great social distance between the two sides and little movement between them. Decisions about admission and discharge are made by authority and the individual has little say in them. The amount of contact with non-institutional life is strictly rationed and is looked upon as a privilege. The inmates sleep, play and work in one place, and an overall rational plan guides all behaviour. Even the smallest detail, such as when an inmate shall bath or cut his nails, may be decided for him. Social experience is reduced to a uniform dullness. The inmate is no longer looked upon as a father, or an employee, or a customer, or as a member of numerous specialised groups, and his ability to play everyday social roles may atrophy from disuse. He does not practise travelling on buses, or spending money, or choosing food or clothes. His relationships with the outside world are reduced to a minimum.

These are features of 'bad' institutions—authoritarian, custodial, and deadening—and they are the reason for the recent reaction against the use of the institution for solving or alleviating social problems. As Titmuss (1959) has pointed out, 'No such swing of opinion away from the *good* institution can be discerned: the effective general hospital for the acutely ill, the public school and other socially approved forms of institutional care. But these have been experienced and remembered only by a minority; for most people institutional life has spelt little besides ugliness, cheapness and restricted liberties.'

Many of the general factors which total institutions are said to have in common may certainly be seen in mental hospitals, and all the features of behaviour and attitudes which make up the syndrome of institutionalism may readily be found among long-stay mental patients (Barton, 1959; Belknap, 1956; Dunham and Weinberg, 1960; Goffman, 1961).

However, there still remains the problem of cause and effect, which a purely descriptive analysis such as Goffman's does not help to resolve. Patients are admitted to mental hospitals for many reasons and it is not obvious, *a priori*, that some of them would not develop in such a way (or in some other way which is equally damaging) if they were not admitted. Indeed some patients look 'institutionalised' at the time of admission. Nor do we know what proportion become 'institutionalised', nor how soon. Goffman has written a brilliant polemic but he is writing within the literary rather than the scientific tradition.

King and Raynes (1968 a) have devised an index, based on Goff-man's ideas, which they have applied to the measurement of 'inmate management' in various residential institutions for the mentally retarded. They distinguished four processes of management in Goffman's account—inflexibility of routine, regimentation, de-personalisation and social distance—all of which were less evident in voluntary or local authority children's homes or hostels than in mental subnormality hospitals. They argued that 'the reasons for the contrasting patterns of upbringing as between the two types of institution are to be found in characteristics of their social structure: the hospitals are hierarchical, over-departmentalised and too highly centralised. They are task-oriented rather than child-oriented'. A house-mother regards playing with the children as a natural part of her job; the nurse sees it as a time-wasting interference with her routine (King and Raynes, 1968 b; Tizard *et al.*, 1966).

It is difficult to be sure that such different institutions as mental subnormality hospitals and voluntary homes do not select children with different characteristics, which might themselves influence the type of social environment provided, but Tizard's experiment (Tizard, 1964), and the current evaluation of new services being carried out by Kushlick (1966), provide more direct tests of the efficacy of alternative methods of dealing with the subnormal.

Studies of general hospitals have also shown that certain aspects of social organisation affect the morale and efficiency of staff and hence, by inference, the quality of a patient's treatment. Revans (1962) found that ward sisters' opinions about senior staff, their attitudes towards student nurses, the stability of qualified nursing staff on the wards and patients' mean length of stay were all signifi-cantly interrelated, in fifteen general hospitals. It is plain enough that 'if a message about a special diet is held up because the ward sister is on bad terms with the dietician, the patient on the special diet is bound to suffer', but studies of this kind are not directly focussed on patients' suffering nor on their clinical condition. A stay of sixteen days in hospital compared with nine days (the range of average stay found at the fifteen hospitals) does not necessarily mean that patients suffer more than moderate inconvenience or discomfort in the hospitals where discharge is delayed. On purely *a priori* grounds it could be argued that a longer stay means more complete treatment.

At any rate, it cannot be taken for granted that a shorter stay automatically means better treatment. Cartwright (1964) interviewed a representative sample of 700 people recently discharged from hospital and documented their discontents. Like Revans, she found much dissatisfaction with the quality of communications, and numerous specific instances of bad organisation, but the patients' overall judgement was favourable. Although mortality rates vary from one hospital to another, especially between teaching and non-teaching hospitals, it has not been shown that variations in staff morale or specific aspects of social organisation are responsible.

The literature on institutions for old people also provides firm evidence that inmates are subjected to unnecessary discomfort and distress, which improvements in social organisation and in the standard of material care could, in the main, prevent. Handicaps have been quantified and social arrangements systematically reviewed (Townsend, 1962).

The student of mental hospitals can see analogies in other institutions and can formulate hypotheses about the likely effects on mental patients after considering what happens to the subnormal or the old or the physically ill once they are segregated from the rest of the community. Nevertheless, large and important questions remain, to which answers cannot be suggested by reference to other institutions or general institutional theory. More help is forthcoming from the specific literature on mental hospitals.

THE SOCIAL ENVIRONMENT OF MENTAL HOSPITALS

There is a particularly rich literature on the history and development of mental hospitals which has been summarised by Kathleen Jones (1954, 1960). The social organisation of mental hospitals during the first half of this century was largely concerned with the safe custody of the inmates at a low cost to public funds. This had not always been the case. The 'moral treatment' practised in many asylums a hundred years earlier was based on principles which would be generally accepted today: for example, the emphasis on early discharge which is now taken for granted in United Kingdom hospitals (Conolly, 1856; Deutsch, 1949; Rees, 1957; Bockoven, 1956; Jones, 1954, 1960). This period was not prolonged. The hall-marks of the era which followed were large and overcrowded hospitals, with a high proportion of chronic wards in which long-stay patients led a restricted and inactive life. Over 60 per cent of the schizophrenic patients admitted remained for at least two years, after which their chance of discharge became very low. There was general pessimism about the outcome of any schizophrenic illness (Brown, 1960a). A legacy which still remains today is that three-quarters of all beds in public mental hospitals are occupied by long-stay patients, most of them suffering from schizophrenia.

At any mental hospital in this country the older members of the staff can recall those days, and vestiges still remain even in the most advanced institutions. At one large hospital which is now well-known for the high quality of the treatment of its long-stay population, the changes in staff attitudes which have taken place are still documented in the shirts issued to the patients. Large red C's are sewn prominently on the front of the oldest shirts. (The C referred to the central store.) On more recent issues this mark is attached at the waist line. In the newest shirts it is relegated to the tail, but it is still present. Even in this hospital there are patients who do not possess a handkerchief, and some wards are still painted in institutional browns and buffs, which have not been changed for twenty years.

The social characteristics of two American state mental hospitals which were primarily custodial in function have been described in some detail by Belknap (1956) and Dunham and Weinberg (1960). The major function was to prevent a mentally ill individual from harming himself or others and to ensure that he could not escape. Routines of supervision and control were developed which would leave nothing to chance—hence the railed airing-courts, the locked doors, the windows that would only open two inches, and the warning whistle that every attendant carried. Given the twin facts of a large patient population and a small inadequately-trained staff, it was inevitable that procedures which were adopted for the control of a few potentially dangerous patients should be generalised to the relatively amenable majority. The same rule of economy applied to many other activities. As Goffman (1961) points out, much time and trouble can be saved 'if everyone's soiled clothing can be indiscriminately placed in one bundle, and laundered clothing can be redistributed, not according to ownership, but according to rough size'.

The movement towards reform took two main lines which at first ran parallel to each other but are now tending to converge. On the one hand, there was an emphasis on rehabilitation and resettlement through the provision of meaningful domestic and industrial roles within an open hospital setting, leading through transitional communities of various kinds to full participation in community life for a certain proportion of patients (Barton, 1959; Bell, 1955; Bennett, Folkard and Nicholson, 1961; Bennett and Wing, 1963; Carstairs, O'Connor and Rawnsley, 1956; Early, 1960; Freudenberg, Bennett and May, 1957; Wadsworth, Scott and Tonge, 1958; Wing, 1960; Wing, Bennett and Denham, 1964). On the other hand, there was an emphasis on early discharge, or the avoidance of admission altogether, in order to prevent the accumulation of long-stay institutionalised patients (Carse, Panton and Watt, 1958; Macmillan, 1958 b).

These methods were empirical and based on a revival of many of the techniques of moral treatment, which had been basically 're-educational'. It is still arguable how far they, rather than the introduction of new drugs such as Reserpine and Chlorpromazine contributed to the dramatic reversal of the long-continued upward trend in mental hospital bed-occupancy, which was first noticed in 1955. It seems probable that the pioneers' use of social techniques began in certain hospitals well before the national swing was noticed in 1955, and the underlying statistical trends must have long antedated the change in overall bed-occupancy. Pharmacotherapy then made it easier to improve social conditions in hospitals where change had not already begun.

Another movement was also extremely influential, although it did not originate in mental hospitals and only later spread to them. Basically, the concept of the 'therapeutic community' consisted in the assumption that patients and staff working together in groups would be able, through the sharing of experiences and feelings, to develop a better appreciation of how disturbed social roles led to symptom-formation and eventually to definition as patients. This understanding, in turn, was expected to enable the patients to modify their attitudes and behaviour even after they left hospital. The concept was first elaborated at length by Maxwell Jones (1952), who subsequently applied it to other settings (1962) and also put it into practice in a small Scottish mental hospital (1968). Martin (1962) and Clark (1964) described their experiences in applying the ideas in mental hospitals. Stanton and Schwartz (1954) provided a more systematic psychoanalytic gloss and this line of development has been carried on particularly at the Yale Psychiatric Institute, where Rubenstein and Lasswell made an analysis in terms of political power-sharing (1966), but did not consider the clinical effects on patients.

The 'therapeutic community' concept is best seen as an ideology rather than as a theory of treatment, although there seems no reason why it should not be formulated in a testable way. There seems to be something about the concept which invites a lack of precision but Rapoport has shown, in a preliminary way, that it is possible to make progress in definition and evaluation. He found that the attitudes of patients (mainly with character disorders or neuroses) at the Henderson Hospital did change while they were there, but that there was no discernible long-term effect (1960).

Freeman, Cameron and McGhie (1958) applied the ideas, in modified form, to schizophrenic patients and demonstrated improvements among some whose handicaps had been thought to be irreversible. Letemendia, Harris and Willems (1967) studied a group of seventy-seven long-stay schizophrenic men in 1959 and again in 1964. Roughly half of the patients had been transferred during this time to a new division of the hospital, run on the lines suggested by Maxwell Jones (1952, 1962, 1966) and Clark (1965), and spent the last three years of the period under these conditions. The measurements were mainly clinical and showed virtually no change in either group over the five-year period. Since no social indices were included it is impossible to know whether transfer to the new division actually did involve any considerable change in environment, and since there was no measure of social withdrawal (probably the best measure of severity in chronic institutionalised schizophrenic patients—see next section) there is no means of knowing whether patients changed on this important variable. Nevertheless, taken together with the results of Clark and Hooper (Clark, Hooper and Oram, 1961; Hooper, 1962), it is difficult to be optimistic about the general effects of introducing a 'therapeutic community' so far as schizophrenic patients are concerned.

Many other studies have been made which enable the authors to claim at least behavioural improvement following social changes in a ward regime. The most obvious successes have come when gross neglect was corrected (this phase was already over when Letemendia's study was started). Ytrehus (1959), Gottfries *et al.* (1968), L. Wing (1956), and others have made this kind of demonstration. More specific effects have been difficult to demonstrate and, when control groups have been used, the results of social measures such as 'habit training' have not been very spectacular. One odd effect, however, has been a common deterioration of patients in the control group (Wing and Freudenberg, 1961). Further discussion of studies which attempted to measure the handicaps of schizophrenics, and the effects of social treatment or rehabilitation, will be found in the next section.

A few systematic comparative studies have been carried out to compare hospitals with different social policies or environments but, as in the studies of general hospitals, it is exceptional for the supposed effects on patients to be measured directly. The book by Jones and Sidebotham (1962) may be taken as an example. Three quite different types of hospital were compared, using as an index of efficiency the 'cost per short-stay patient-week'. The apparently most expensive unit provided the most intensive treatment and care, turned over its short-stay patients most rapidly and had the best follow-up results when the samples were matched for sex, age, diagnosis and social class. But Jones and Sidebotham correctly point out that in-patient costs are an inadequate measure of efficiency since the cost of un-employment and other hidden costs must be taken into account. They were not able to find a way of doing so, but by making an estimate and multiplying it by the average length of stay they arrived at a cost per patient which was lowest at the hospital with the highest apparent costs. The authors are well aware that their calculations are based on far too many assumptions (particularly about the equivalence of patients admitted to the three hospitals) to carry much weight, and they claim no more than that they 'have provided a beginning to the study of a very large subject'. This claim is justified but it is also important to point out that the evaluation of different types of social policy and social structure can only be properly undertaken when there are adequate measures of morbidity in patients and relatives. Administrative indices such as length of stay, staff–patient ratio, re-admission rate or cost-per-patient-week are valueless in themselves.

Another work may be mentioned in some detail because it, too, uses length of stay as an index. The core of the book by Ullman (1967) is the description of a careful study designed to test the hypotheses that the size and staffing ratios of Veterans Administration psychiatric hospitals would each be related to indices of outcome, such as length of stay and prospect of staying for two years or more. The hypotheses were indeed confirmed but it was also shown that other factors, such as a relatively high financial budget spent on administration, a high pressure of applications for admission and the presence of an active family care programme were important intervening variables, so far as size was concerned; in fact size alone did not contribute anything once they had been taken into account.

The economic implications of these findings are well discussed. What is less acceptable is the starting assumption that length of stay is in any way significant as a measure of severity of illness. There is overwhelming evidence against this. Not only were many long-stay patients unnecessarily detained in hospital in the old days, but many severely-ill patients are now being discharged after a very brief stay. Indeed, many British hospitals are now down to what must surely be the minimum stay, but they cannot all be regarded as of equal quality. Some countries must do without any mental hospital beds at all. It may well be found, even in a relatively well-serviced area, that the substitution of small and highly-staffed hospitals for mental hospitals may lead to an *increase* in the length of stay of newly-admitted patients, although the quality of care is improved. Data from the Camberwell Register, for example, indicates that this is occurring in London (Wing, Wing and Hailey, 1970). Oram and Knowles (1964) demonstrated, as Ullman has done, that pressure for admission reduces recruitment to long-stay status, and there are numerous other studies to show that the presence of alternative facilities, or a simple change in attitude on the part of doctors, can result in rapid changes in length of stay, or sudden discharge of long-stay patients. Thus the conclusions concerning administrative or financial problems are well worth taking into account, as are those of Jones and Sidebotham. To generalise from administrative indices to morbidity, however, is to make them carry more weight than they will bear.

THE EFFECTS OF MENTAL HOSPITALS ON LONG-STAY
SCHIZOPHRENIC PATIENTS

Barton (1959) states the hypothesis that features of the institution such as loss of contact with the outside world, enforced idleness, bossiness of staff, loss of personal friends and possessions, drug treatment, poor ward atmosphere and loss of prospects outside the institution lead to a syndrome of 'institutional neurosis' which he defines in some detail. Each of his terms is further specified and it is a pleasure to see hypotheses stated so clearly. Although he is not specifically dealing with schizophrenia he thinks that much of the 'end-state' said to be a characteristic of that disease is a product of social forces. A much less clear-cut concept is that of the 'social breakdown syndrome'. Gruenberg and his colleagues have shown that empirically defined behaviours correlated with social withdrawal and hostility in psychiatric patients have become less frequent and last for shorter periods when they do occur, compared with former years. They argue that this clinical improvement is likely to be due to the reorganisation of psychiatric services which took place during the same period, resulting in a shorter stay in hospital for many patients, and out-patient support and supervision after discharge. Both the 'social breakdown syndrome' and its putative causes ('traditional attitudes towards the mentally ill') are very complex and no attempt is made to test hypotheses concerning more specific causes and effects. Nevertheless, an important demonstration has been made, one of the first of its kind (Gruenberg, 1966; Wing, 1967; Zusman, 1966).

Goffman's work has already been mentioned. He does not use conventional psychiatric terminology and tends to explain patients' behaviour solely in terms of their reactions to the social environment. Other sociologists have also made a deliberate attempt to see how far they can go in explaining the phenomena of mental illness without recourse to biological explanations (Mechanic, 1968; Scheff, 1963, 1964).

At the other extreme it is almost impossible to find a contemporary psychiatrist who believes that the end-state seen in chronic schizophrenic patients is entirely due to deterioration inherent in the disease process. Nevertheless, the concept of schizophrenic deterioration is deeply ingrained in psychiatric thought even though it is difficult to demonstrate it (Foulds and Dixon, 1962).

Three types of factor are clearly likely to play a part in determining how a person reacts to long incarceration in an institution: the social pressures which are brought to bear; the susceptibility or resistance of the individual to these pressures, and the length of time over which the pressures act (Wing, 1961).

Many of the negative features of 'total institutions' have been present in mental hospitals, at least up to ten years ago, and most patients who had been continuously resident for two years in 1960 would have been exposed to them. In addition, dietary deficiencies and the physiological effects of prolonged underactivity must be considered (Kety, 1959). The most positive pressures—resocialisation, re-education, rehabilitation, somatic treatments of various kinds and psychotherapy—have been applied unevenly at different hospitals and were introduced much later in some institutions than in others.

Susceptibility to the social pressures of the old-fashioned mental hospital must also vary a good deal. Patients who have not built up strong ties in an outside community through marriage or work or family or other interests; those who are vulnerable because of poverty or age or social position; those who have never been concerned with problems of personal liberty and decision-taking; those in whom social relationships induce anxiety or discomfort and who prefer a social environment where interaction can be minimal—all these may have an increased liability to admission, and their chance of discharge later on may be reduced. Thus there may be, for various reasons, a state of susceptibility to institutionalism which is present when the individual first enters the segregated community, so that, at its most extreme, a person may show dependence on the institution, and apathy about leaving, very shortly after admission (Ellenberger, 1960). The essence of the concept of institutionalism, as so far discussed, is that long-term exposure to the social pressures of the institution has brought about a change in the individual's behaviour and attitudes; but the limiting case occurs where such behaviour is already present in embryo before admission. If a great many such people are admitted, the apparently high prevalence of 'institutionalism', compared with that in another community, may be misleading.

So far as schizophrenia is concerned there is another problem— how far the typical symptoms of the illness (in which shallowness of emotional response and lack of motivation are common symptoms even when the patient has never been admitted to hospital) can be distinguished from the aspects of behaviour and attitudes which are said to be characteristic of institutionalism. Schizophrenic patients, by reason of their numbers and prolonged residence, acquire, transmit and partially determine the peculiar culture of the hospital community (Sommer, 1959). The problem of institutionalism in mental hospitals becomes, therefore, in large measure, the problem of the long-term management of schizophrenia.

Thus it is important to establish whether institutional procedures cause deterioration in schizophrenic patients. Such deterioration might take place either in symptomatology, or in aspects of behaviour and in attitudes which could reasonably be regarded as part of a syndrome of institutionalism even in people who were not ill (for example, dependence on the institution, apathy about leaving, lack of interest in events outside, lack of competence in extramural activities, resignation towards the institutional mode of life, and so on). Since, logically, either of these two sets of factors may vary independently of the other, any investigation into the effects of prolonged institutional pressures should differentiate between them as clearly as possible, though some overlapping cannot be avoided. (In particular, apathy and flatness of affect, unrealistic ideas about the future and delusions, must overlap.)

Finally, there is the problem of length of exposure to the institutional pressures. A short-term deprivation of liberty, even with complete and perhaps humiliating change of routine, is unlikely to have much lasting effect on the average individual (for example, during a brief stay in a general hospital) unless there is some kind of susceptibility. On the other hand, many years in a 'maximum-security' prison, exposed to a rigidly monotonous regime which allowed no opportunity for individual responsibility in deciding everyday behaviour, would surely affect most people in some way, though a number of resistant individuals would undoubtedly be found. Edith Bone, for example, gave an account of seven years spent in solitary confinement. If the liveliness of her writing is anything to go by, she can have suffered very little diminution of personality during this time, and indeed she found an extraordinary variety of ways in which to keep her mind alert and occupied. In general, however, one would expect that the longer a person had been exposed to a deadening routine the more likely he would be to show traits of institutionalism. On the other hand, specific environmental pressures of various kinds might accelerate or slow down the process of change, and determine its direction. Since a long-term study of changes in behaviour and attitudes over many years has obvious practical difficulties, it might appear sensible to compare individuals at one point in time who had been resident in a total institution for varying periods. There is a serious objection to this method, however, unless the effect of selection can be allowed for. Not only may individuals succumb immediately to institutional pressures (with an exacerbation of symptoms or the appearance of institutionalised behaviour patterns) but there may be a selective effect of certain social characteristics, such as marital and occupational status, on length of stay. This is certainly true of schizophrenic patients in mental hospitals (Norris, 1956; Brooke, 1957). Brown (1960*b*) has shown that schizophrenics who were visited during the first two months after admission in 1950 had a much greater chance of leaving hospital than those who were not. No doubt a similar selective effect could be found in those who were apathetic on admission, which could partly account for any higher proportion of apathetic patients in the longer-stay groups.

THREE THEORIES LINKING SCHIZOPHRENIA AND THE
SOCIAL ENVIRONMENT

In such a complex field there can be no simple theory from which to predict how schizophrenic patients will react in various social environments. However, it is possible to see three linked theories which cover a large part of the ground.

The first concerns the differentiation of three main types of disability from which patients may suffer—'premorbid', 'primary' and 'secondary'. The second theory concerns the way in which 'primary' disabilities vary under different types of social pressure. The third is concerned with the origin and modification of secondary handicaps. None of these theories reaches a high level of abstraction and all contain elements which are speculative, questionable or vague, but each allows the construction of testable hypotheses.

1. *Handicaps in schizophrenic patients*

The various factors which may hinder the resettlement of a schizophrenic patient can be classified into three large groups:

(*a*) disabilities which are present before the overt onset of schizophrenia, such as a poor education, a difficult personality, a physical disability or low intelligence;

(*b*) disabilities which are basically part of the illness, such as incoherent thought processes, delusional motivation or catatonic slowness or apathy;

(*c*) 'secondary' handicaps which are not part of the illness itself but which have accumulated because the patient has been ill, and because of his own and other people's reactions to the illness.

These types of handicapping factor have been described in detail elsewhere (Wing, 1963) and only a brief account will be given here.

(*a*) 'Premorbid' handicapping factors have frequently been described in schizophrenic patients. Hare (1956), for example, showed that patients who later became schizophrenic tended to move out of a family setting and to seek a socially isolated area of town before the first onset of florid symptoms. Dunham (1965) confirmed this tendency to 'drift'. Goldberg and Morrison (1963) showed the same thing for occupational decline. Even when one particular occupation was taken, for example that of clerk, Wardle (1962) was able to show that future schizophrenic patients tended to have less responsible and less socially active work than future manic-depressive patients. The effect continues after the onset of the psychosis. Brown (1960*b*) showed that visiting during the early days after admission to hospital was associated with length of stay, and Brooke (1957), Cooper (1961), Hollingshead and Redlich (1958), Norris (1956) and Ødegaard (1946, 1953) have shown that factors like class and marital status also affected chances of discharge, irrespective of diagnosis. Thus certain handicapping or supporting characteristics may be present or absent before overt disease develops and profoundly affect the outcome when it does.

For our immediate purposes it is not necessary to consider whether some 'premorbid' impairments are actually early manifestations of a disease process before it becomes clinically manifest, though this seems quite possible. The two basic types of symptom which we

2

describe in the next section might very well have their precursors which lead to a poor premorbid performance of various social roles.

(*b*) The concept of 'primary' handicap is taken from general medicine, where specific dysfunctions can be defined in terms of theories of normal functioning. For example, the normal limits within which blood sugar or haemoglobin can vary are well established. Chronic dysfunctions defined in these terms are likely to give rise to obvious 'primary' disabilities which, again, can be classified in various ways (Piercy Report, 1956). It is more difficult to define the 'primary' disabilities in schizophrenia and other psychiatric conditions since the relevant theories of normal functioning are not yet developed, but certain motor difficulties (such as slowness), and psycho-physiological abnormalities (of skin conductance, for example, or two-flash threshold) have been described and confirmed. It is useful as a working arrangement to take certain of the chronic symptoms of schizophrenia as an indication of the presence of primary disabilities, although they are often elaborated and complicated by other elements in the patient's personal and social life. Most chronic symptoms can be classified under the headings used by Kraepelin and Bleuler—disorders of affect and of association. We shall refer to these two types as 'negative' and 'florid' symptoms.

Negative symptoms include social withdrawal, flatness of affect, poverty of speech, lack of initiative, slowness, under-activity and a low level of motivation. The work reviewed by Venables (1960, 1967, 1968) leaves little room for doubt that a substantial biological component is involved. Ratings of social withdrawal are highly correlated with measures of autonomic and cortical activity such as skin potential, and two-flash or two-click threshold. There is a close relationship between skin potential, social withdrawal and a simple subclassification of chronic schizophrenic patients (Venables and Wing, 1962). Social withdrawal seems to be a useful measure of the severity of schizophrenia.

Florid symptoms include delusions, hallucinations, incoherence of thought and speech, over-activity and various forms of odd behaviour. The relationship to possible psycho-biological dysfunctions is less evident than in the case of negative symptoms, though certain symptoms, such as thought echo, thought insertion and perceptual distortion which, in the early stages, are often described very clearly, without any delusional elaboration, suggest that such dysfunctions may be present. In any case, there is no doubt of the socially handicapping effects of chronic negative or florid symptoms.

Although we shall deal with these two groups of symptoms separately, we do not wish to exclude the possibility that flatness of affect and social withdrawal are a protective reaction which helps to cope with the cognitive impairment. There is some evidence for this in our earlier work (Brown *et al.* 1962). Venables and Wing (1962) also found that patients with incoherence of speech as a predominant symptom were best classified with patients with poverty of speech, and that social withdrawal tended to be just as great. Patients with coherently-expressed delusions, on the other hand, seemed to form an independent group. We shall therefore consider the various symptoms separately.

(*c*) A patient suffering from any chronic illness is liable to develop 'secondary' handicaps which do not arise directly out of the disease process, although they would not have occurred if he had remained well. There are two main types. In the first place, there is the patient's personal reaction to being ill, depending not only on the nature and severity of the disease, but on his previous personality, social attitudes and experience of illness. Secondly, there is the reaction of the social groups, general and local, in which the patient plays a part, and upon whose goodwill his conditions of life may depend. If these two kinds of reaction are favourable, even a severe primary disability may not hinder a patient from achieving a successful resettlement. If they are adverse, even a mildly handicapped patient is likely to remain unsettled.

In any particular case, the three types of handicap fuse together to give one clinical picture, but in order to plan a course of rehabilitation most successfully, it is necessary to separate the various elements and to be aware of the different kinds of environmental factor which can cause deterioration or improvement in them. The other two linked theories give some guidance in this respect.

2. *Effect of the social environment on 'primary' disabilities*
The second theory concerns the way in which the social environment affects 'primary' disabilities. There is good evidence that severe negative symptoms can quite suddenly improve or get worse under

different conditions of social stimulation (Wing and Freudenberg, 1961). A more gradual change has also been postulated (Wing and Brown, 1961). It may be suggested that many schizophrenic patients are biologically vulnerable to under-stimulating environments and liable to respond by a marked increase in social withdrawal. Even a symptom like flatness of affect, according to this theory, is not necessarily immutable but, in many patients, will be dependent on the social milieu. Observations of this kind presumably also explain the disappearance of catatonic motor phenomena from mental hospitals (Achté, 1961) even before the introduction of the new drugs while, at the same time, warning that they could just as readily return if social and biological therapies were withdrawn.

The most evident example of an exacerbation in florid symptoms is the 'admission crisis' (Brown *et al.*, 1966; Smith, Pumphrey and Hall, 1963; Wing *et al.*, 1964) which precedes such a high proportion of admissions to hospital and is usually based on a sudden increase in intensity of delusions or hallucinations which affects the patient's behaviour. Such exacerbations are also well-known in long-stay patients. Stone and Eldred (1959) observed the re-emergence of delusions in two patients who had been free of florid symptoms for many years, shortly after they had been transferred to a special treatment ward. Wing, Bennett and Denham (1964) also found, in a study of a rehabilitation unit, that six out of forty-five long-stay schizophrenic patients showed an unmistakable exacerbation of symptoms during the first week. Five of these adverse reactions took place in patients who had not been adequately prepared for the course.

Brown and Birley (1968) have made a systematic investigation of social precipitating factors in our current study of schizophrenia in south-east London. They were concerned only with patients whose attack was of sudden onset which could be dated to within a week. They defined very carefully the kind of social events they were interested in, such as changes in health, residence or social role either of the subject or of a close relative, and then, by means of interviews with patients and relatives, they estimated the frequency of such events in each of the thirteen weeks preceding the onset (which might have been the first onset of the condition or a sudden relapse following a remission). They went to some trouble to get adequate controls from the general population of the area. While the proportion of subjects in the general population who experienced social events within the defined categories remained fairly steady at about 20 per cent per three-week period, there was a markedly higher frequency (60 per cent) in the three-week period preceding a schizophrenic breakdown. This was still true when only those social events were considered which were extremely unlikely to have been dependent upon some earlier, but undetected, change in the patient's clinical condition. Breaking an engagement would be an example of an event which might conceivably be due to some prior change in the patient, even one which had not been noticed by anyone or reported by himself. Witnessing a serious street accident, and having to appear in court to give evidence, would be an example of an event which is likely to be independent of possible schizophrenic symptoms. The two classes of event showed the same time relationship to onset.

Brown *et al.* (1962) showed that knowledge of the degree of emotional relationship between a key relative and a schizophrenic patient at the time of discharge from hospital gave very useful information about clinical prognosis during the subsequent year and, in a recent replication of this study, we have been finding a fascinating interaction between longer-term social 'stresses' such as the degree of tension in a household, phenothiazine-taking and frequency of precipitating factors (Brown and Birley, 1968; Birley and Brown, 1970).[1]

Thus there seem to be at least two fundamental processes at work. On the one hand, an under-stimulating social environment tends to increase symptoms such as social withdrawal, passivity, inertia and lack of initiative. This process is obviously seen best in the old-fashioned type of mental hospital but it can quite easily occur in the community as well. On the other hand, there is the tendency to break down, with an effusion of florid symptoms, under conditions of social over-stimulation. This second process is most frequently seen outside hospital but it can certainly also be seen within it. These are general statements and the two processes sometimes vary together. The complexity of the psycho-physiological processes involved has

---

[1] There is much indirect epidemiological evidence that migration and other social factors may precipitate attacks of schizophrenia, at least in susceptible individuals, but there are alternative explanations in terms of various kinds of social selection, and the work will not be reviewed here.

been described in detail by Venables (1968)—for example, the most withdrawn schizophrenic patient is found to be over-aroused—and it would be premature to suggest how the variation in the social environment produces changes in symptomatology. Nevertheless, the sketch of a theory is discernible and depends on the assumption that negative symptoms are a protective reaction against the cognitive impairment. When the patient is allowed to withdraw, he does so, and the process can easily go too far. When he is not allowed to withdraw, but faced with what seem to be impossible demands, the underlying thinking disorder becomes clinically manifest in florid symptoms. The optimum environment is presumably well-structured, with clear lines of behaviour laid down and a neutral type of social stimulation which does not lead to emotional over-involvement: both thought disorder and withdrawal are then minimised.

3. *Effect of the social environment on 'secondary' disabilities*

A quite different theoretical approach is required when considering 'secondary' handicaps. This concept is somewhat similar to that described by Lemert (1951) as 'secondary deviation' but it is used from a medical point of view. For Lemert, 'primary deviation' occurs during the early stages of socially unusual behaviour, when the individual can still manage to rationalise it in terms of a socially acceptable role. 'When a person begins to employ his deviant behaviour or a role based upon it as a means of defence, attack, or adjustment to the overt and covert problems created by the consequent societal reaction to him, his deviation becomes secondary.' How long the assumption of normality can be kept up varies in different individuals and Lemert does not sufficiently emphasise this point. Schizophrenic patients are particularly likely to resist a societal definition of their behaviour as abnormal. They tend to lack insight and to be over-confident about their chances of achieving a reasonable level of social, occupational and domestic performance (Wing *et al.*, 1964). However, if deviant acts are disrupting, repeated and socially visible, the societal reaction becomes correspondingly severe and the individual *has* to adjust to it. Once the patient is admitted to hospital, particularly if the chances of discharge are remote, the expectations of staff and other patients become paramount. The longer the patient stays, the less likely is he to practise everyday social roles and any ability that he originally had may atrophy from disuse. The patient, who originally has no intention of staying in hospital (Wing *et al.*, 1964), gradually changes his attitudes and eventually may not wish to leave (Wing, 1961). 'Institutionalism' of this kind is a special case of the development of secondary handicaps. If patients remain in the community, without becoming long-stay, the processes of societal control are relatively less intense. Nevertheless, probably everyone who is handicapped because of illness develops secondary disabilities. Hewitt (1949) found that physically disabled men who were unemployed tended to do nothing but walk the streets and read the papers in public libraries. They frequently had pathological attitudes of resentment, depression and anxiety. Hewitt came to the conclusion that 'the attitude of mind of the disabled man is the largest single factor in determining the prospects of future employment'.

Such attitudes reflect not only the clinical effects of the illness and the disabled person's view of himself, but the opinions towards him which important people in his environment adopt. We did not find (contrary to the general view) that schizophrenic patients' relatives are specially rejecting, and parents, particularly, tend to be very tolerant, even in the face of extremely difficult behaviour, but their attitudes do not always reflect back to the patient the image of himself which would be most helpful to his progress. Wives and husbands are less tolerant, and the divorce rate of married schizophrenics is three to four times that in the general population (Brown *et al.*, 1966). Olshansky, Grob and Malamud (1958) have shown how important the attitudes of employers are.

The process of acquiring secondary handicaps can be described in terms of reference group theory, which is also useful for deriving hypotheses about how to change attitudes. The application of reference group theory can be illustrated by an experiment at an Industrial Rehabilitation Unit in London, to which handicapped people of all kinds were sent, mostly with physical disabilities but quite a large proportion with psychiatric handicaps. Two-thirds of the entrants lacked confidence in their ability to find and hold down a reasonable job. Some of them acquired this confidence during a short course at the Unit—on the whole, they were the ones with most constructive attitudes to start with. The others remained unconfident.

Those who gained confidence tended to be successful in finding work when they left; the unconfident ones tended to be unsuccessful (Wing, 1966 b). Festinger's adaptation of reference group theory was invoked to explain these results (Festinger and Kelly, 1951; Festinger, 1957). People who wish to join a particular group will tend to adopt the attitudes and behaviour characteristic of this group. In therapeutic terms, the problem is to provide a social setting where confidence is a group-approved attitude and where it is visibly successful in that confident people get reasonable jobs. This is precisely the setting of the rehabilitation unit. Those with reasonably constructive attitudes can take advantage of such a social environment and this included some with schizophrenia.

There is a larger problem, however, in psychiatric rehabilitation, in that many patients with long-term disabilities (and, in particular, many schizophrenics) have already acquired unconstructive attitudes and the straightforward procedures of the rehabilitation unit are not sufficient to help them. They may indeed already be *over*-confident. Rehabilitation is a very long process with such people, although the basic theories are the same. It has to proceed by very small steps. That attitudes to work, for example, can change in chronic schizophrenic patients, and that such change can alter the social prognosis, has in fact been demonstrated (Wing, 1960; Wing, Bennett and Denham, 1964).

Even so, there will be a group of schizophrenic patients who do not respond to any of these measures, because their apparently 'secondary' handicaps are, in fact, 'primary'. For example, an attitude of indifference to work or family may, in some patients, be a negative symptom with an underlying biological basis which can only be reduced to a certain extent by environmental treatments. Similarly, unrealistic attitudes may be part of a delusional system which is unresponsive to social measures. Techniques of rehabilitation have two aims in such cases—to prevent the development of further secondary handicaps so that advantage can be taken of any clinical improvement that does occur, and to provide a series of sheltered environments in which the patient's assets will be maximised and his disabilities will be least evident.

AIMS OF THE PRESENT STUDY

The present study was primarily concerned with the adverse effects on schizophrenic patients of a prolonged stay in three selected mental hospitals and with the ways in which these effects could be counteracted and prevented. Aspects of all the three theories mentioned above are involved and it is impossible to detail every hypothesis that was tested. It should be emphasised, however, that the intention was to find causes, not just associations. We therefore measured the social environment, not in general, but as it impinged upon each patient individually.

To take the social factors first, we expected to find that a number of different aspects of the social environment would be associated together to form a milieu of 'social poverty'. The longer a patient stays in hospital the more intense (if that is the right word) his experience of social poverty is likely to become. Hospitals with a high reputation for rehabilitation and resocialisation will be characterised by less social poverty, but the hypothesis should still hold true. Energetic reform should decrease the amount of social poverty.

So far as clinical measurements are concerned, we expected to find a syndrome of 'clinical poverty' predominant in a representative sample of the schizophrenic patients at the hospitals. The worse the social poverty experienced by a patient the worse his clinical poverty should be and, therefore, the hospital with the most social poverty should contain the most patients with clinical poverty. Florid symptoms were not expected to vary very much with social poverty or length of stay or between hospitals. If social poverty were decreased at any of the hospitals, clinical poverty should decrease concomitantly, but only in those patients whose social conditions had improved. Florid symptoms might be expected to get worse if vigorous techniques of resocialisation were introduced without prolonged preparation.

The main hypotheses concerning secondary handicaps were that attitude to discharge from hospital would depend on poverty of the milieu and, independently, upon length of stay. Since specific measures to change attitudes to discharge were not expected to be introduced for large numbers of patients, it was assumed that these attitudes would not change over time or that they should, if anything, become rather more unfavourable.

We did not attempt to say in advance why *social* changes would take place but, since detailed and systematic social measurements would be made on several occasions, we hoped to be able to describe what occurred, and to throw some light on the reasons for any changes, which might lead to hypotheses about the process of reform in mental hospitals.

We hope that it is fairly clear by now that this study formed one part of a programme of research into the nature of the interaction between social and clinical events; an interest which forms the main basis of social psychiatry.

2

THE DESIGN OF
THE STUDY AND METHODS
OF MEASUREMENT

Design of the study

The three hospitals were selected for study because they seemed to differ markedly in social conditions and administrative policies and their staffs were likely to collaborate actively and closely. The characteristics of the hospitals are described in detail in Chapter 3. It was decided to study female patients, first in order to check previous work which had been concerned with men only, and secondly because, in these particular hospitals, the contrasts between women's wards seemed likely to be greater.

The matron of each hospital was asked to supply a list of names of all female patients in the hospital together with age, length of stay, diagnosis and ward. A random sample was taken from each ward in Netherne Hospital and Severalls Hospital of 120 female schizophrenics who had been resident more than two years and were aged under 60. Twenty of these acted as 'spares'. All the 73 women in Mapperley Hospital with these characteristics were selected. The diagnosis was checked from the case-notes and at interview with each patient. Four patients at Netherne Hospital, none at Mapperley Hospital and one at Severalls Hospital had to be replaced on diagnostic grounds. In addition a sample of case-notes at each hospital was checked to make sure that long-stay patients with other diagnoses were not in fact schizophrenic by the criteria used in this study— very few extra cases were discovered in this way and no change of procedure was necessary.

After several months of developmental work, investigators spent a week at each hospital interviewing patients and staff and collecting information. Severalls was visited in March 1960, a few weeks after the new physician superintendent had taken up his appointment, Netherne in June 1960, and Mapperley in September 1960.

Further surveys were carried out two years later at Mapperley and Severalls and all three hospitals were again visited after four years.

[27]

Finally, certain rating scales were again completed in January 1968.

The two investigators did not discuss their material as it was being collected, nor did they refer to previously collected data. By the time of the third survey, however, the psychiatrist recognised some of the patients and sometimes remembered the approximate pattern of earlier ratings. There could be no question of blind ratings, and unconscious bias of various kinds cannot be eliminated. However, the same investigators carried out a follow-up study of schizophrenic patients admitted to the same three hospitals in 1956, and did not confirm their expectations in one important respect, so that they do not have a 'set' to discover what they are looking for, nor an obvious bias in favour of demonstrating that social conditions which seem preferable, *a priori*, actually are making a difference to patients, in practice (Brown *et al.*, 1966).

Methods of measurement

CLINICAL CONDITION

Ratings based on standard interview, and clinical classification

The technique of this very simple interview has been described else-where (Wing, 1961). On the basis of questions about attitude to discharge, plans for the future, life in the hospital, general knowledge and symptomatology, four symptoms are rated on a 5-point scale:

> flatness of affect
> poverty of speech
> incoherence of speech
> coherently-expressed delusions

A rating of 1 means that the symptom is not present; 2 that it is only suspected to be present because of information from case-notes; 3 that it is present in moderate degree; 4 that it is markedly present; 5 that it dominates the interview—the patient shows no affect, is mute or almost mute, speaks fluently but completely incoherently, or can talk of nothing but delusions (see Appendix 2.1).

These ratings may be used on their own or they may be combined to give a very simple classification into seven subgroups:

1*a*. No symptoms at interview (rating of 1 or 2 on all scales).

1*b*. Moderate symptoms only (rating of 1, 2 or 3 on all scales).

1*c*. Moderate speech symptoms only (rating of 3), but rating of 4 or 5 on affect.

2. Predominant symptom is coherently-expressed delusions (rating of 4 or 5).

3. Predominant symptom is incoherence of speech (rating of 4 or 5).

4. Predominant symptom is poverty of speech (rating of 4).

5. Mute or almost mute (rating of 5 on poverty of speech).

This system of rating, with or without the categorisation, has been used by Catterson, Bennett and Freudenberg (1963), Morgan (1967), Calwell, Jacobsen and Skarbek (1964), Hamilton (1964), Hamilton and Salman (1962), Storey (1966), Philip and McKechnie (1969), Skarbek and Hill (1967), Collins and Dundas (1967), Hunt (1967), Ekdawi (1966) and Venables and Wing (1962).

Catterson, Bennett and Freudenberg (1963) and Willis (1964, personal communication) made surveys of all the male and female schizophrenic patients who had been in their hospitals (Netherne and Stone House) for more than two years and were aged 60 or less. The distributions are shown in Table 2.1 (p. 195), which gives some idea of the variation that is to be expected between hospitals, using this method. It may be compared with Tables 5.10 (p. 213) and 7.10 (p. 231). The mean S.W. scores shown in Table 2.1 represent the ratings of social withdrawal made by nurses describing the behaviour of schizophrenic patients under their care. The way the scores are derived is explained below in the section on ward behaviour.

The validity of the distinction between moderately and severely affected individuals was shown by Wing (1960) who found that only the former group was likely to benefit from a course at an Industrial Rehabilitation Unit. The usefulness of the distinction was demonstrated by Morgan (personal communication) who found that he had selected predominantly moderately handicapped individuals for his rehabilitation hospital. His results can therefore only be generalised to this group. The same is true of the work of Wing, Bennett and Denham (1964). On the other hand, Wing and Freudenberg (1961) demonstrated a useful technique of social treatment for severely handicapped long-stay schizophrenic patients.

Ward behaviour

A simple ward behaviour rating scale, to be completed by nurses, was described by Wing (1961), and is presented as Appendix 2.2. Factor analysis of the ratings of two separate sets of schedules demonstrated two main factors: one represented by items correlated with social withdrawal, the other by items such as over-activity, and laughing to self, designated 'S.E.' ('Socially embarrassing behaviour'). Since each item can be scored 0, 1 or 2, the maximum score on S.W. is 16, and on S.E. is 8.

The S.W. score was found to be reliable both between raters and between occasions, in the preparatory work, and by other investigators (e.g. Philip and McKechnie, 1969). The S.E. score is much less reliable since the behaviours measured are very variable.

A useful indication of reliability of the two forms of measurement (interview and 'S.W.' rating scales) can be obtained from studying their relationship. The figures given by Catterson, Bennett and Freudenberg (1963) and Willis (1964, personal communication) are presented in Table 2.1 (p. 195).

These patterns of scores are clearly very similar and they compare very well with the results of the present study. In measuring change, it can be estimated that the S.W. score would need to drop by some 5 points if a patient were reclassified from clinical group 5 (mute or almost mute) to clinical group 4 (predominantly severe poverty of speech), and by another 3 points for a reclassification to clinical groups 1*a* or 1*b* (symptoms of moderate severity only). A decrease in S.W. score is likely to be a more sensitive measure of improvement, therefore, but improvement in clinical symptoms is likely to be a more stable index.

A further check was possible from data collected at Netherne Hospital by Venables who had rated many chronic schizophrenic patients on an 'activity–withdrawal' and a 'Paranoid–Non-paranoid' scale (Venables, 1957; Venables and O'Connor, 1959), according to which they could be subdivided into four groups—active non-paranoid, active paranoid, withdrawn paranoid and withdrawn non-paranoid. These groups are roughly equivalent to subgroups 1, 2, 3 and 4+5 of the present classification. Out of 57 patients rated by both techniques, 40 (70 per cent) were placed into equivalent categories (C = 0·74).

Venables and Wing (1962) showed that psycho-physiological measurements also differentiated reliably between the various categories. The relationship between social withdrawal and biological indices such as skin potential and 'two-flash threshold' is fully discussed by Venables (1968).

Many other variables are related both to clinical classification and to ward behaviour (particularly the S.W. score). Catterson, Bennett and Freudenberg (1963), for example, showed that industrial output and general knowledge were highly associated.

In summary, the two techniques constitute reliable and valid measures of clinical condition in long-stay schizophrenics and probably represent, in part, biological abnormalities. They can be used as crude measures of severity of clinical condition, of chances of discharge and of level of social functioning within the hospital. The S.W. score presumably also contains an attitudinal component from the nurse (see Wing and Freudenberg, 1961) and is therefore less valuable than clinical classification in looking for associations with other nurse-rated variables.

Attitude to discharge

All patients were asked a series of questions:

How do you like it in hospital?

Would you like to leave?

How strongly do you feel about it?

(If wants to leave.) Do you want to go as soon as possible or would you be prepared to wait a bit?

For how long?

Have you anywhere to live?

Would your people be glad to welcome you?

What about supporting yourself?

(If wants to stay.) How long do you want to stay?

Do you want to leave eventually?

Would you like to make your home here permanently?

(All patients.) If the doctor advised you to leave (stay) would you agree?

On the basis of the answers, each patient's attitude to discharge was classified as follows:

1. Strong desire to leave hospital.

2. Desire to leave hospital but qualified in some way (e.g. 'As soon as I can find a place to live or a job'), or unrealistic.

3. Patient ambivalent about leaving, gives contradictory replies, or is very vague about plans for the future. Nevertheless, the answer does include a statement that the patient wants to leave.

4. Patient seems indifferent about leaving or staying, or so vague that no attitude can be rated at all.

5. Patient definitely, or on balance, wishes to stay in hospital. (N.B. In the correlational analysis, codes 1, 2 and 3 were combined and given a score of 1, the remaining codes being scored 2.)

The results of a previous study using a similar technique were described by Wing (1962). The reliability, when ratings were checked against self-ratings by the patient after being shown a card with three alternatives, was satisfactory. Some examples are given in Appendix 6.1 (p. 112).

Freeman, Mandelbrote and Waldron (1965) have used more extended interviews with long-stay schizophrenic patients in Littlemore Hospital, Oxford, and found that the desire for discharge became less frequent the longer the patient had been in hospital. However, the more extended the interview, the more difficult it is to fit the patient into categories 1 or 5.

Catterson, Bennett and Freudenberg (1963) found that 38 per cent of their comparable sample (both sexes) had some desire to leave hospital (33 per cent in the present study) and 28 per cent wanted to stay (29 per cent in the present study).

The problem of changing attitudes of this kind are fully discussed by Wing (1960) and Wing, Bennett and Denham (1964).

Therapeutic drugs

Since somewhat different drugs were used at the three hospitals it was impossible to use the daily dose in milligrams to evaluate the place of drug treatment. Each drug was therefore scored in terms of arbitrary units which were chosen so as to be approximately equivalent to each other. The equivalents, in milligrams, of one unit of the commonest drugs were as follows:

Chlorpromazine	100	Perphenazine	4
Promazine	100	Prochlorperazine	12½
Reserpine	1	Trifluoperazine	5
Thiopropazate	5		

A similar procedure was used for anti-depressant drugs and sedatives but the details are not specified since very little difference was found between the hospitals or over time, and these drugs were not very commonly used.

SOCIAL CONDITIONS
Personal possessions

A female research assistant (usually a nurse from the hospitals concerned) made an inventory of all the personal possessions of each patient in the series (whether initially provided by the hospital or privately), by interviewing the patients and nursing staff and checking with the patient the contents of lockers and wardrobes. Strict ownership was not required; continuous and sole use was considered sufficient to define personal possession. For example, if a dress or towel was marked with a patient's name, and returned to the same patient each time after laundering, it was classed as personal property. An inventory of seventy articles of clothing or objects for personal use was used as a check list. Some results are summarised in Table 6.3 (p. 218).

These lists have an interest which goes far beyond the possibility of quantifying possessions in general (important as this obviously is). Performance of a female role requires the availability of accessories such as handbags and make-up, the use of potentially dangerous instruments such as needles, scissors and mirrors, and the expression of individuality in clothing. Morgan and Cushing (1966) have discussed the importance of personal possessions to long-term patients.

Time budget

The sociologist interviewed the appropriate ward sister (and often another nurse) about each patient in the series and, where necessary, the patient herself. The purpose of the study—and particularly the need to obtain accurate and frank accounts of patient's behaviour and staff opinions—was explained. The confidential nature of the enquiry was emphasised. The list of patients in the sample who lived on the sister's ward was then read out, and information was collected as to how each one had spent her time on the previous day. Considerable detail was required about all activities, from the time of getting up until going to bed; what time the patient rose, who woke her, whether she dressed herself and how long this took, the details of her toilet, whether she made her bed, how long she waited for breakfast, and so on through the day. If there was any doubt on sister's part, the patient herself, or another nurse, was interviewed. This information was often very easy to collect because of the high predictability of much of the patient's behaviour. It was not unusual for the sister to be able to describe the exact position and even posture of a patient at any time during the day. Some patients, for example, would stand against the same ward radiator for the whole day, except at meal-times. Other staff, for example the occupational therapists, were asked to describe activities which took place away from the ward. These data were categorised in various ways, and the number of hours per day spent in each activity was calculated (see, for example, Table 5.4, p. 207).

Nurses' opinions about patients

The ward sister, and one other nurse, were separately asked by the sociologist thirteen standard questions about each patient's ability to cope with certain everyday activities and responsibilities. These included whether she could visit the local shop without asking, whether she could do useful work in the hospital, or go out with a male patient. Details of the questions are given in Chapters 5 and 6 and in Appendix 2.3. Intercorrelations between the two nurses' scores in 1960 were 0·70 (Netherne), 0·64 (Mapperley) and 0·45 (Severalls). See also Table 2.2 (p. 196).

Patient's occupation

The nurses who filled up the questionnaire about patient's ward behaviour were also asked to complete sections concerning recent occupation, contact with the outside world, and physical treatment. The questionnaire is presented in Appendix 2.4.

The occupation section was scored as shown on p. 35.

The correlation between occupation score and the number of hours doing nothing (calculated from the time budget obtained by the sociologist) was −0·64 in 1960, and −0·51 in 1964.

		Score
Work outside hospital	2e	15
Industrial work	3f	10
Unsupervised work	2d	9
Work in service departments	2c	8
Domestic work	2b	7
Competent ward work	1d	6
Daily occupational therapy	3e	5
Supervised working party	2a	4
Reliable washing up, etc.	1c	3
Occasional occupational therapy	3b, c, d	2
Very little ward work, no occupational therapy	1b, 3a	1
Unemployed	1a, 3a	0

Contact with the outside world

The questions asked are detailed in Appendix 2.5. The scoring procedure was as follows:

		Score
Goes home regularly and has visitors	2a, 1a or 1b	15
Goes home regularly. No visitors	2a, 1c	13
Goes home occasionally and has visitors	2b, 1a or 1b	11
Goes home occasionally. No visitors	2b, 1c	9
Doesn't go home. Visited regularly	2c, 1a	6
Doesn't go home. Visited occasionally	2c, 1b	4
Doesn't go home. No visitors	2c, 1c	3

This score was modified, if necessary, as follows:

		Score
Town parole	3d	+2
Ground parole	3c	−1
Not allowed outside ward except in supervised working party	3b	−2
Not allowed outside ward except under individual supervision	3a	−3

Ward restrictiveness

The day-to-day management of certain of the female wards was considered in detail. All wards in which more than 20 per cent of the patients were long-stay schizophrenics under 60 years of age were considered. In 1960, this applied to eight wards at Netherne, five at Mapperley, and eight at Severalls. These wards contained 83 per cent of the 273 patients studied. Forty items were covered by direct questioning, of which five were subsequently discarded because they were repetitive. Each of the remaining thirty-five items was scaled, the total possible score being 50 points (representing maximum restrictiveness). The items are shown in Appendix 2.6. Thirteen were concerned directly with restrictions on the movement of patients, such as locking of ward doors, the necessity for staff permission to leave the ward, and the seclusion of patients in side-rooms. The remaining twenty-two items were concerned with more general rules and routines—restrictions on the use of the bathroom, regulations about personal clothing, access to the ward kitchen, and so on. The two parts of the schedule gave very similar results, and the scores were therefore combined. In designing scales for each item, attention was paid to the proportion of patients affected by a regulation (it was only rated highly restrictive if a large majority was involved), and whether it was applied with discretion. For example, on some wards each patient's hair was washed in the weekly bath, as a matter of course, although, as one patient pointed out, she had been to the hairdresser on the previous day. Such indiscriminate application of the rules was scored more heavily for restrictiveness.

Some further questions were asked about facilities—such as the number of lockers available on each ward.

There was likely to be a tendency for nurses to present their wards in the best possible light. However, most staff members were pleased to talk and surprisingly frank in what they said about hospital life. A number of checks were possible, since the interviewer was on the ward for many hours and could observe, for example, whether the baths were screened and how many lockers were available. Any inconsistencies were pointed out and discussed.

At the time of the surveys in 1962 and 1964 a similar procedure was applied. The wards considered were often different to those used in 1960 and no direct correlation of scores is therefore possible.

OTHER MEASURES

In addition to the measures mentioned above, information was collected about the patient's age, date of admission, date of first admission, height, weight, father's occupation, and marital status on admission.

The case-records were also abstracted in order to obtain some picture of the clinical course since the patient had been in hospital. The notes varied very considerably, both in quality and in quantity.

Very little other information could be systematically obtained for all patients, but we did, of course, make notes about conversations with numerous staff members and patients, and about our everyday observations during the time we were living in the hospitals.

CONSTRUCT VALIDITY

Evidence concerning the reliability and validity of some of the measures has already been considered. The face validity of most of the instruments is high—it is fairly obvious what they 'mean'. However, their construct validity can also be ascertained, that is, the extent to which they are correlated together in clusters which form meaningful entities. Information concerning clinical classification and S.W. score has already been presented. Other aspects of construct validity are discussed in Chapter 4.

APPENDIX 2.1

Scales for rating four schizophrenic symptoms

1 Flatness and incongruity of affect

1 No evidence
2 Indirect evidence only (e.g. case-notes)
3 Occasional episode of definite flatness or incongruity, but mainly appropriate affect
4 Affect mostly inappropriate or flat, but occasionally appropriate
5 Complete flattening. No affect unless incongruous

2 Poverty of speech

1 No evidence
2 Indirect evidence only (e.g. case-notes)
3 Definite vagueness, stereotypy, repetitiveness or wandering, but interview relatively intact.
4 So vague, wandering, repetitive or stereotyped, that interview almost impossible
5 Mute or almost mute

3   Incoherence of speech

  1 No evidence
  2 Indirect evidence only (e.g. case-notes)
  3 Definite incoherence, but rest of interview little affected
  4 Definite incoherence, interfering markedly with rest of interview
  5 Practically nothing coherent

4   Coherent delusions

  1 No pre-occupation evident
  2 Indirect evidence only (e.g. case-notes)
  3 Some evidence of coherently expressed delusions, but these have little force now. Little active pre-occupation
  4 Evident active pre-occupation, but can give attention to other matters
  5 Can hardly attend to anything else

APPENDIX 2.2

Ward behaviour scales

Please consider this patient's behaviour during the past week only, even if it was not typical of his or her usual condition.

There are three items in each section. If one of the items describes behaviour which has occurred in the past week, please place a tick against it in the column on the right. There should be only one tick for each section. Please read all three items before making your choice.

Item 1: Slowness of movement

(2) Usually extremely slow to move, e.g. took very much longer over a meal, or dressing, or walking across the ward, than other patients
(1) Showed periods of extreme slowness of movement as in (2), but at other times was not slow to move
(0) Speed of movement normal

Item 2: Under-activity

(2) Stood or sat in one place all the time, with little movement. Even with encouragement was very difficult to get moving
(1) Showed periods of extreme under-activity as in (2), but at other times was not under-active
(0) Showed no marked under-activity

Item 3: Over-activity

(2) Usually extremely over-active or restless, e.g. paced rapidly up and down, became excited, talked or sang loudly or wildly, etc.
(1) Showed periods of extreme over-activity as in (2), but at other times was not over-active
(0) Showed no marked over-activity

Item 4: Conversation

(2) Was mute or almost mute
(1) Said a few words, e.g. in reply to questions, but was usually silent
(0) Ordinary conversation

Item 5: Social withdrawal

(2) Never mixed socially with anyone, even when encouraged to do so
(1) Was socially withdrawn and solitary, but would mix a little with others if encouraged to do so
(0) Normal social mixing

Item 6: Leisure interests

(2) Showed no interest in anything. Did not watch television, read newspapers, play games, etc., even when encouraged to do so
(1) Showed very little interest, but could be persuaded to watch television, read papers, join in games, etc., for a while
(0) Showed normal spontaneous interests

Item 7: Laughing and talking to self

(2) Frequent episodes (once a day or more often) of laughing or talking out loud—not just constant smiling
(1) Occasional episodes of laughing or talking out loud, but these did not occur every day
(0) No such episodes noted

Item 8: Posturing and mannerisms

(2) Adopted odd or uncomfortable postures, or made bizarre movements, every day
(1) Behaved as in (2), but less often than every day
(0) No such behaviour seen

Item 9: Threatening or violent behaviour

(2) Struck some person, or destroyed some article (e.g. clothing, window, crockery, etc.)
(1) Was threatening in manner, or verbally abusive, but did not strike anyone
(0) No such behaviour seen

Item 10: Personal hygiene

(2) Was incontinent on at least one occasion during the week
(1) Needed raising at night, or escorting to lavatory during the day, in case of incontinence, but was not actually incontinent when this was done
(0) Needed no escorting or raising and was not incontinent

Item 11: Personal appearance

(2) Needed to be shaved (if male), washed or dressed fully at least once during the week

(1) Could shave, dress and wash, but needed supervision with tie, buttons, etc., or would be slovenly in appearance
(0) Needed no supervision of this kind. Maintained reasonably neat appearance without prompting

Item 12: Behaviour at meal-times
(2) Needed spoon-feeding at least once during the week
(1) Did not require spoon-feeding, but had to wear bib, or needed supervision because of faulty table manners
(0) Normal behaviour at meal-times

APPENDIX 2.3

Nurses' attitudes

1	Could this patient do useful work for the hospital—such as laundry, typing or domestic work—if it were available?	*Yes*	*No*
2	Could this patient be allowed to bath when she likes, without asking permission?	*Yes*	*No*
3	Could this patient be allowed to possess matches?	*Yes*	*No*
4	Does this patient appreciate money; for example, would she appreciate being paid 10s. instead of 5s.?	*Yes*	*No*
5	Could this patient be quite free to visit the local shops when she likes?	*Yes*	*No*
6	Could this patient be allowed to go out with male patients (e.g. to the local cinema)?	*Yes*	*No*
7	Should this patient definitely be helped to buy her own clothing?	*Yes*	*No*
8	Could this patient be allowed to possess scissors?	*Yes*	*No*
9	Could this patient look after the money she might earn?	*Yes*	*No*
10	Need this patient be certified?	*Yes*	*No*
11	Could this patient manage to do some kind of work outside but while living in the hospital?	*Yes*	*No*
12	Could this patient be discharged now, if a job was found and she had a suitable place to live?	*Yes*	*No*
13	Does this patient need to stay in a locked ward?	*Yes*	*No*

APPENDIX 2.4

Patients' occupations

Please consider the patient's main work during the past month. Tick one item in Section 1 *or* Section 2 (not in both) for all patients: but do not count occupational therapy—there is a separate section (3) for this.

Section 1: No work outside the ward or ward garden
(a) Unemployed

(*b*) Contributes very little towards ward work (e.g. a little polishing or dusting)

(*c*) One to three hours' ward work daily at a fair level (e.g. reliable washer-upper)

(*d*) Four or more hours' competent ward work daily. The ward would be difficult to run without this patient

Section 2: Work outside the ward

(*a*) Member of a supervised working party (e.g. on grounds, drive, etc.)

(*b*) Work in sewing room, main kitchens, laundry, cafeteria, staff quarters, other wards

(*c*) Work in service departments (e.g. stores, bakehouse, engineer, shoemaker, coalcart, etc.)

(*d*) Individual work on farm or gardens (not a member of a working party)

(*e*) Work outside hospital

Section 3: Occupational therapy

Please tick any item which applies:

(*a*) None

(*b*) One or two hours daily, in ward

(*c*) Three or four hours daily, in ward

(*d*) Occasional visit to O.T. Department

(*e*) Goes to O.T. Department every day

(*f*) Does industrial contract work

APPENDIX 2.5

Contact with the outside world

Please tick one item in each section.

Section 1: Visiting during past six months

(*a*) Visited once a month or more often

(*b*) Visited less often than once a month

(*c*) Not visited during the past six months

Section 2: Visits home during past six months

(*a*) Visited home once a month or more often

(*b*) Visited home less often than once a month

(*c*) No visit home during past six months

Section 3: Parole status

(*a*) Not allowed outside ward unless under escort

(*b*) Only allowed out when in supervised working party

(*c*) Ground parole (not under supervision)

(*d*) Town parole

If constant supervision is needed, please state why:
    May try to escape
    May wander away
    May be aggressive or threatening
    May be destructive
    Appearance may be frightening to others
Please state any other reason below:

APPENDIX 2.6

Items of ward restrictiveness scale

A. *Movement*

1 Time outside door of ward locked
2 Locking of internal doors (except store rooms and nurses' rooms)
3 Time patients went to bed
4 If and when patients were locked out of ward
5 If and when patients were required to inform nurse when leaving the ward
6 Whether free to visit hospital shop without permission
7 Whether free to visit hospital entertainments without permission
8 Whether free to visit local shops without permission
9 Entries in 'seclusion book' in last month
10 Number of patients 'secluded' in side-rooms on previous night
11 Restrictive clothing on the ward
12 Whether there was a railed 'airing-court' attached to the ward
13 Whether patients were kept waiting at the conclusion of meals

B. *Other restrictions*

1 Access to bed during the day
2 Whether bathing was permitted only on certain days
3 Whether a key (to taps or door) was used as a means of supervising bathing
4 Times at which bathroom was opened
5 Whether a nurse was present whenever any patient was bathing
6 Whether patients were allowed to do their own laundry
7 Whether hair of patients was washed by the nursing staff
8 Whether beds were made by nurses or a few ward workers
9 Whether patients were allowed more than one article of hospital clothing at a time (e.g. dress)
10 Whether patients had ready access to their own private clothing
11 Whether patients could change into their private clothing without permission
12 Whether the same items of hospital clothing were returned to patients after laundering
13 Whether there was a free choice of the amount of sugar and milk in tea

14 Whether patients were free to switch on and control TV set or wireless
15 Whether patients were allowed to use the ward kitchen for minor tasks (e.g. making tea)
16 Whether patients were free to smoke at any time outside the dormitory
17 Whether patients could possess matches
18 Whether there was a formal means of making complaints (e.g. ward meetings)
19 Whether current newspapers were supplied
20 Whether *Radio Times* was supplied
21 Whether patients were able to lock lavatory door
22 Whether baths were screened from other patients

3

THE THREE MENTAL HOSPITALS

The medical, nursing and occupational-therapy staff at all three hospitals were very willing to collaborate in the study. Much of the material collected was descriptive as well as quantitative and some of it will be presented in Chapter 8. However, the book would be incomplete without a general account of the hospitals themselves and, in particular, of the policies and intentions of the most influential people—the physician superintendents. We therefore asked Dr Barton, Dr Freudenberg and Dr Macmillan to write a brief account of their hospitals and the policies they had consciously followed in trying to structure the social environment. We specially asked them to add a note on priorities, since it is perfectly plain that no one could attempt to make every department of the hospital function in an optimum way with the limited resources available. Their accounts are not edited, but some standard information on obvious indices such as catchment area and bed-occupancy is given first.

Mapperley Hospital, built in 1880, had 940 beds at the end of 1959 and had reduced its numbers by 300 during the previous eight years. The main hospital had been divided into a male and a female side in 1960. On the ground floor of the female side there were two main admission wards and a sick ward for medical and surgical treatment and a ward for elderly patients. On the ground floor of the male side there were two main admission wards and a sick ward for medical and surgical cases. On the first floor on both sides the wards were used as hostel wards, rehabilitation wards and community centres for day patients (there were 16,700 day patient attendances during 1960, at all units). One of the long-stay wards was almost entirely self-running, there being only one part-time nurse present during the day. The long-stay wards were looked after medically by part-time general practitioners under the supervision of a consultant psychiatrist. In addition there was dormitory accommodation on the second floor.

St Ann's Hospital, containing male and female admission wards and a children's unit, and St Francis Hospital—a psycho-geriatric unit—contained no patients in the present series, nor did Porchester

House—a hostel in the grounds of the main hospital. Another hostel, Park House, situated about a mile from Mapperley did contain several patients in the series.

There have been no locked wards at Mapperley Hospital since October 1952. In 1960, three prefabricated occupational therapy units were in use at the main hospital.

The hospital group provides services for a population of 401,000, comprising the City of Nottingham, two adjacent county suburban areas and one other county urban area about nine miles distant. The area is an industrial one and was largely developed in the nineteenth century. Long terraces of red brick cottages are characteristic in the centre of the city, and newer developments on the outskirts consist largely of council housing. A third of the housing is publicly owned and only a quarter 'owner-occupied'. In extent, it is much smaller than the other two areas, and nowhere more than nine miles from the hospital, as compared with thirty miles at Netherne and forty-five miles at Severalls. Of 1,664 patients admitted to Mapperley during 1960, 1,301 were from the city, 316 from the county of Nottingham, and 47 from elsewhere.

Severalls Hospital was opened in 1913 and had 1,590 patients at the end of 1959. There had been a reduction of 130 beds during the previous eight years. The physician superintendent had recently retired after twenty years' service, and the new chief doctor had been in office six weeks at the time of the first survey in April 1960. The hospital had been passing through a period of change, though the process had been taken further in the male than in the female wards. Progress had not been as rapid as at the other two hospitals. However, throughout the institution the major features of an earlier period—side-rooms used for seclusion, electro-convulsive treatment and sedation used instead of occupational therapy and skilled supervision to control disturbed behaviour—were beginning to disappear. Padded rooms were not in use and were about to be removed. The railings round the airing-courts were being taken down. Much remained to be done, compared with the other two hospitals, but this hospital was not by any means the worst that could have been chosen. There were ten female wards in the main building occupied by 60 per cent of the long-stay patients. The rest were in seven nearby villas. One of these had been devoted to the care of private patients before

National Health Service days and it still retained a genteel and comfortable atmosphere which was in marked contrast to the rest of the hospital. The wards and villas catering for long-stay patients tended to be larger at Severalls than at Mapperley or Netherne; only 2 out of 14 had fewer than 50 beds, compared with 11 out of 19 at Netherne and 4 out of 7 at Mapperley.

The hospital is situated on the outskirts of Colchester, a town of 65,000 people fifty-four miles from London. It serves an East Anglian population of just under 550,000, almost one-third of whom live in local government rural districts—compared with 11 per cent at Netherne. Just over 100,000 live in Dagenham, thirty-nine miles away, and the remainder in scattered urban areas including Chelmsford (50,000), twenty-two miles away, and the New Town of Harlow (53,000), forty miles away. Unlike the Netherne area, none of the districts served by the hospital is London-centred. Even in Dagenham, which is an outlying part of the London conurbation, a smaller proportion of the employed population travels to work in Central London than from any part of suburban Surrey served by Netherne. Nearly two-fifths of the housing is publicly owned, largely because of the concentration of public housing in Dagenham and Harlow. About two-fifths is 'owner-occupied'.

The former physician superintendent, in a note contributed to the booklet prepared for the Jubilee celebrations of the hospital in 1963, ended with a pertinent comment concerning the earlier history of the mental health services: 'As we dig out and reject—as indeed we must—much that was built into the pattern of fifty years ago, we may perhaps avoid too arrogantly and publicly giving thanks to Providence that we are not as others were, and perhaps have the wit to perceive something worthy of respect, rather than ridicule, in the lessons of the Past.'

Dr Russell Barton, the physician superintendent, who succeeded in 1960, has published a book called *Institutional Neurosis* (1959).

Netherne Hospital had 1,860 beds at the end of 1959. There had been a reduction of 150 beds during the previous eight years. The physician superintendent himself supervised, in 1960, the two villas which housed the most severely ill chronic schizophrenic patients. There was an active rehabilitation policy throughout the hospital under the direction of Dr Freudenberg (who was seconded to the

Ministry of Health from 1961 to 1964), and Dr D. H. Bennett (who left in May 1962), and special methods were used to help long-stay patients to become self-supporting outside. There was a separate short-stay hospital (Fairdene), a day hospital in Carshalton and full out-patient services at general hospitals throughout the area. There were twelve female wards in the main building. Eight of these (one of them locked) were occupied by 40 per cent of the long-stay female population. A further 30 per cent were cared for in six villas, two of which were special rehabilitation units (each containing both male and female patients). One was designed to prepare moderately handicapped long-stay patients for discharge, the other to treat a group of severely disabled patients. The remaining 30 per cent were housed in a separate building, a former workhouse, about ten miles away from the main hospital. Most of them were over 60 years of age. The amenities in this unit were considerably poorer than in the rest of the hospital and the social atmosphere was quite different. There was difficulty in recruiting nurses to work there. The hospital lay in rural surroundings, at about the point where the southern suburbs of the London conurbation merge into the rural and outlying urban districts of Surrey. The hospital serves a population of some 650,000 people, of whom just over three-quarters live in one or other of the suburbs (Carshalton, Sutton and Epsom) and the remainder in the two towns of Reigate and Dorking (12 per cent) or in the surrounding local government rural districts (11 per cent). It is a prosperous area in which much of the housing was developed after the First World War, and 60 per cent of it is 'owner-occupied'. With the exception of the rural districts, and Reigate and Dorking, a high proportion of the employed population works in Central London.

Journeys to the hospitals

Because of the varied areas in which the hospitals were situated, travelling to and from hospital had quite different meanings for patients and relatives. In Nottingham, in 1960, a journey from the centre of the city to the hospital by bus took about fifteen minutes and cost 6*d.* each way. Journeys from outlying estates took longer and cost more, but never lasted as much as an hour and rarely cost as much as 2*s.* each way, and because of the excellent service from the centre to the hospital never involved a long wait at a bus stop.

At the other extreme, to go from Harlow to Severalls Hospital took three and three-quarter hours, including almost an hour waiting at or walking between bus stops. The journey involved travelling on five different buses, cost 14s. 4d. each way, and was typical of many in the Severalls area: a journey from Dagenham, for example, cost over 10s. each way and took more than three hours on four different vehicles. Sometimes it was possible to speed the journey by taking a train. From Chelmsford one could, for example, reach Severalls in a little over an hour, but the cost was rather more than by bus (Anne Race, *Severalls Hospital Annual Report*, 1960).

In the Netherne area a typical journey from Epsom took nearly two hours, including half an hour's wait in Reigate, and cost 3s. 8d. each way. A journey from Purley lasted only a quarter of an hour and cost 1s. From Leatherhead the journey took nearly two hours and cost 3s. 11d. each way.

MAPPERLEY HOSPITAL

by Duncan Macmillan, O.B.E., B.Sc., M.D.,
F.R.C.P.E., D.Psych.

Mapperley is situated in the north-east corner of the City of Nottingham, and is responsible for the mental health services of that city and of some surrounding urban areas. The population for which it has to provide services increased from 311,000 in 1954 to 394,000 in 1956, because of acceptance of an additional three county urban areas in order to alleviate the difficulties being encountered by the neighbouring county mental hospital. By 1965 the population had increased to 406,000.

The in-patient services of the hospital have been reduced from 1,328 beds in 1948 to 651 in 1966. This total includes all the beds in the main mental hospital, three admission units for men, women and children situated a mile away, two hostels, the addiction unit, and the psycho-geriatric hospital three miles away.

The reduction in the number of beds was a steady, gradual process, and was a planned procedure with specific objectives and a definite order of priority. There were four main phases, the first of which was the development of an extensive system of out-patient services, and of community activities based on integration with the local authority services, combined with the provision of adequate early treatment in-patient facilities. The second objective was the establishment of hostels and hostel accommodation and of sufficient day hospitals to provide the necessary supportive care and treatment for patients in the community requiring economic rehabilitation or social resettlement. The third major objective was the provision of a system of geriatric prevention, day care, and early treatment, but I shall make only a brief reference to this, as I have recently described it elsewhere (Macmillan, 1967).

There was a definite degree of overlapping in the measures designed to attain these three initial objectives. The fourth and last, which is still in process of development, was the active in-patient rehabilitation of the remaining long-term in-patients and of those long-term patients in the community who periodically required admission for in-patient rehabilitative measures.

The in-patient aspect of the first objective was to provide a sufficient number of admission units to furnish appropriate environment and proper classification for early treatment, with reasonable individual amenities and without overcrowding. This necessitated reduction in the number of beds in these units, so that each patient received adequate individual care and treatment.

These admission units were closely linked with and formed one aspect of the scheme of community mental services which had been in operation since 1946, and also operated in close liaison with the out-patient services which had been developing since the early 1930s. The initial diagnostic clinics are held mainly in the general hospitals of the city and also in the out-patient department situated in close proximity to the early treatment admission units. Psycho-therapeutic sessions are carried out separately, chiefly in our own out-patient department, and the after-care clinics are held in accommodation adjacent to the in-patient admission units. The preventive clinics include those for marriage guidance, delinquency and epilepsy.

In child psychiatry the out-patient clinics are organised by the children's psychiatric consultant who is also in charge of the child guidance centres of the local education authorities, the children's in-patient unit, and their day hospital.

The Mental Health Department of the City of Nottingham was established in 1946, and took over the functions of the previous Mental

Hospital and Mental Deficiency Committee. Its objective was to unite under one administration the out-patient treatment of mental illness, in-patient mental hospital treatment, the after-care of mental patients, the community care of mental patients and mental defectives, the in-patient treatment of mental defectives, social psychiatry with all its measures for the prophylaxis of mental illness and for the education of the public in such matters, and 'the mental health of the city generally'.

The difficulties occasioned by the National Health Service Act of 1948 were surmounted, and an integrated scheme was devised, in order to overcome the administrative division between the hospital services and those of the local health authority, which has continued as the integrated hospital and community mental health service which is in operation today.

The emphasis of the service is placed on prevention and early treatment with the objective of intervention in the psychiatric situation, whenever possible, before a serious and long-lasting breakdown in mental health has become established.

As a result of this policy more than half the time of the senior psychiatric medical staff of the hospital has been spent in domiciliary and out-patient work. The total resources of the medical and nursing staffs of the mental hospitals in England and Wales are limited, and it is, accordingly, not possible to implement at one and the same time all the objectives of an ideal mental health service. In our case we have concentrated on prevention, early intervention and early treatment. There are many arguments which could be brought forward in support of this policy. Perhaps they could be summarised in the statements that a stitch in time saves nine, and that, whenever possible, avoidable mental suffering should be alleviated.

When faced with the choice between concentrating our limited available resources on early intervention or on rehabilitation of the long-term psychotic in-patients, the choice was made of the former. It seemed pointless to concentrate on the final stages of an illness, and not make every effort instead to endeavour to prevent the illness from reaching that stage. In the case of schizophrenia the objective is to be able to intervene at the stage when the illness is suspected, but a firm diagnosis is not yet possible, and co-operation and a degree of insight are present. The response is variable, and it is difficult to evaluate statistically the effect of this approach, but clinically one is convinced of its value.

From the practical point of view the results obtained from an equivalent use of psychiatric staff resources in rehabilitating long-term schizophrenic in-patients are limited and partial. Another forceful argument is that if early community measures and out-patient treatment are not combined with active early in-patient treatment, the proportion of schizophrenic patients becoming long-term in-patients must tend to be greater.

It should be made clear that the above statements are not intended in any way as arguments against the desirability of the active rehabilitation of long-term schizophrenic patients, but merely indicate the alternatives with which one is faced in the decision of how best to deploy limited hospital resources.

IN-PATIENT UNITS FOR SHORT-STAY PATIENTS

Excluding the admission units for geriatric patients, the children's unit, and the addiction unit, there are now eight admission units in the hospital, four for each sex, each with numbers varying from 18 to 31, and a total number of 197 beds. Another two admission units are almost completed, and this will increase the number of admission unit beds to 234.

Each of these units discharges its patients directly back to the community and has its own community programme which includes its after-care clinics, domiciliary after-care social visitation, contact with general practitioners, and use of the day hospitals.

The psycho-geriatric hospital is situated in the grounds of the Nottingham City Hospital three miles away from the main hospital and has five ordinary admission wards, three female and two male, each of 20 beds. There are in addition beds available for the use of geriatric day patients when required. Another female ward of 20 beds admits patients for short-term geriatric prophylaxis. One ward of 20 beds is being used for prophylaxis as a mixed ward, providing facilities, when required, for the admission of husband and wife. The remaining ward of 20 beds is being used as an assessment unit for the joint use of the general hospital geriatrician, the local authority welfare services and ourselves.

There are also three female geriatric wards in the main hospital with a total of 72 beds, and beds for the admission of geriatric day patients when required.

DAY HOSPITAL AND HOSTEL SERVICES

The next major undertaking in the evolving process of the in-patient services was the conversion of previous long-stay wards into day hospitals and into hostel accommodation.

Two hostels are administered and staffed by the hospital, one for schizophrenic male patients and one for female patients. Two female wards are run on hostel lines, and male patients are accommodated, as required, in various wards, working in the community under hostel conditions.

The major recent development in the hospital has been the expansion of day hospital treatment from a very small beginning in 1958. During 1965 there were 71,932 day attendances. In addition to its short-term functions as (1) an expansion of out-patient treatment, (2) a substitute for admission, and (3) a provider of after-care, and the important role which it plays in geriatric psychiatry and in children's psychiatry, it is now accepted by us as an essential adjunct to the care and treatment of the long-term psychotic patient in the community.

The day hospital units are now eight in number, four of which, two geriatric and two non-geriatric, occupy four former in-patient wards, and two are day industrial therapy units, of which one is a new purpose-built unit with 100 places, and the other is in the female hostel.

In the psycho-geriatric hospital a geriatric day hospital has recently been established, and in the main mental hospital a rehabilitation ward is being converted into another day unit to provide supportive resettlement treatment. These eight units provide over 350 day places with over 400 day attenders; in addition a few patients come as day patients to their previous admission wards when the consultant considers this advisable.

The amount of care and treatment required by day patients approximates to that necessary for in-patients. Laundering, hairdressing, bathing, dentistry, and provision of clothing are some of the services which are essential components of a day hospital service, if these patients are to be helped to make progress.

In contrast to this, the patients in the considerable number of beds in the hostel and hostel wards require much less attention than formerly. We have found that they do best with a minimum of nursing staff when caring for themselves and one another.

A separate geriatric day centre administered by the local health authority, Nuffield House, provides also a most useful service of prophylactic day care for the elderly.

Day hospital treatment of the long-term schizophrenic patient

Our experience of the day treatment of the long-term psychotic patient in the community has been that it requires reinforcing either by economic rehabilitation or by social resettlement or by both.

ECONOMIC REHABILITATION

The new industrial therapy day unit at the hospital has a section of an outside factory working in it, and is a self-contained unit with its own canteen. Before attending it, patients have a trial period doing industrial work in one of the sections of the occupational therapy department.

The other industrial therapy day unit, designed solely for female attenders, is sited in the female hostel, and has a day nursery for their children.

A sheltered workshop, planned to work in close association with the new industrial therapy unit, still awaits the approval of the Ministries of Health and Social Security.

It has been our experience that schizophrenic patients who are unemployed in the community and do not attain economic independence tend to remain static unless they have intensive rehabilitation by means of industrial therapy under conditions approximating to those of an outside factory.

Social resettlement

Another group of long-term psychotic day patients are unable through their greater psychiatric disability to attain an economic working level, but are able to appreciate living in the community and can attend at the hospital for therapeutic group activities.

These patients require much help with their problems of accommodation and social re-adjustment, and in order to assist them a small

Department of Social Resettlement has been established. The Social Resettlement Officers, in addition to finding accommodation and giving help and guidance in solving the initial financial problems, keep in touch with the patients and their landladies, and continue to help them in the community. The resettlement staff work in close co-operation with the industrial therapy organisation, with the hospital social workers, and the mental welfare officers, as well as with the psychiatrists and nursing staff. The local health authority is working in close liaison with the hospital in this problem of resettlement, and has designated a senior officer of the mental health department to co-ordinate their activities, and to compile a register of landladies.

Transfer or admission to the hostels or hostel wards of the hospital is the first step in the economic resettlement or maintenance of the patient in the community. Our experience has been that a small number of beds are sufficient for short-term patients. Schizophrenic patients require a longer period of hostel stay if subsequent relapse is to be avoided, and will continue to create a need for most of the remaining hostel beds in the hospital.

We found that two types of accommodation are required in the community. The first may be termed 'rehabilitative boarding houses'. In these the patients are helped by the social workers and mental welfare officers, usually on a short-term basis, until they become economically and socially independent. The second may be termed 'supportive community hostels', and are required for the long-term care of those patients who are unlikely to become self-supporting. The resettlement officers pay regular domiciliary visits in order to help with their problems, and at present are looking after approximately eighty former patients in this way in nine boarding houses in the city. Re-admission to the hospital from both types of accommodation is arranged promptly as required.

IN-PATIENT REHABILITATION

The fourth stage in the evolution of the in-patient services of the hospital is one on which we are still engaged, and is the development of active rehabilitative services in five wards, two female and three mixed. The number of patients in them is still excessive, varying from 18 to 48, with a total of 168, and they are not yet functioning fully as therapeutic units.

In the mixed rehabilitative wards definite progress has been made with the therapeutic community approach, organised by one of my consultant colleagues and a senior nursing officer so as to include also those day patients who require long-term community supportive treatment, and also schizophrenic patients requiring admission from the community service for a period of in-patient rehabilitation.

One of the female wards now has an active therapeutic programme in operation, but less progress has as yet been made in the rehabilitation of the long-term schizophrenic female patients.

A Hospital Employment Bureau Committee organises all the arrangements for the occupation of in-patients, and also of those day patients who are not in the industrial therapy organisation. This committee has a consultant psychiatrist as chairman, and has representatives from all sections of the staff of the hospital. They define the work groups, assess the occupational facilities in the various departments of the hospital, place the patients in the most suitable work groups, and build up the patients' work records.

It is planned to reduce the number of beds in the rehabilitation wards to 98 in five units, one of which will be gradually converted to day treatment. This process, which has already commenced, will depend upon the response of the patients to the rehabilitative measures and on the provision of suitable boarding-house accommodation in the community. This is organised by the social resettlement officers as the patients become ready for it, and rehabilitation is then arranged on a day patient basis as required. The process will be a slow and gradual one, and will probably take one to two years to complete.

DISCUSSION

I have described the evolving process in the in-patient services of this hospital in some detail, to explain how the hospital resources were directed initially to the development of out-patient services, of domiciliary community services, of day hospital services with associated economic rehabilitation and social resettlement, and then of active in-patient rehabilitative measures for the remaining long-term patients.

These in-patients are now a relatively small group, a number of whom are becoming geriatric in their needs. They have been kept under constant review with a view to the possibility of return to the community, and are patients whose links with the community have been completely severed and in whom the psychotic process has proceeded so far that economic rehabilitation and social resettlement have not yet proved possible.

The smallness of the group is shown by the fact that only about seventy patients satisfied the criteria for the survey instead of the hundred desired.

Now that it has proved possible to develop more active rehabilitation without impairing the preventive, early treatment, and community aspects of the hospital service, one is impressed by the change in the atmosphere in these wards. The change in attitude is evident in staff, patients, and voluntary helpers. A Patients' Social Activities Co-ordinating Committee is playing a major role in this development, and is composed of representatives from the wards, the League of Friends, the W.R.V.S., the nursing and medical staff, the administrative staff and the occupational therapy department.

In the mixed wards the grouping of the long-term in-patients with the day patients and the periodic re-admissions produces an atmosphere of hopefulness and encouragement which, I consider, would be lacking if the rehabilitative group activities were limited purely to a long-term in-patient group.

We regard these activities, which have yet to reach full fruition, as another essential stage in the process of transforming the hospital into an active treatment centre in which every bed has an active therapeutic function. This is a slow process in the case of the long-term in-patient schizophrenic.

The hospital is now a focal centre from which many services extend out into the community and into which many others are received. We have found that the long-stay needs, which previously used most of the beds in all mental hospitals, can now be met with a very much smaller number of hostel beds, using a fraction of the previous hospital bed complement for active rehabilitation.

At present Mapperley Hospital provides a full range of treatment, resettlement, and rehabilitation with 1·6 beds per thousand of the population served. The extent of the services is illustrated by the fact that during 1965 there were 1,864 admissions, 20,690 out-patient and domiciliary attendances, and 71,932 day attendances.

For further information see Macmillan, 1956, 1957, 1958*a*, 1960, 1961, 1963.

SEVERALLS HOSPITAL

by Russell Barton, M.B., M.R.C.P., D.P.M.

The principal changes in Severalls between 1960 and 1964 are aimed at accomplishing the following objectives: to improve patients' contact with the outside world; the provision of useful occupation to every patient; the adoption of an attitude of encouragement and friendliness to each patient without foolish concessions; an emphasis on the quality of personal life of patients; a reduction of drugs; the provision of a friendly, permissive ward atmosphere with the provision of wardrobes, chests of drawers and individual territory for every patient; assistance with work, accommodation and friends outside hospital. These principles of care were outlined in *Institutional Neurosis* (Barton, 1959) which was distributed to every ward by the H.M.C. in January 1960.

These objectives were examined by medical and nursing staff in a series of lectures, group discussions, ward meetings and refresher courses organised by the physician superintendent at first but increasingly by nursing staff. They have continued ever since.

To prevent patients getting lost by transfer from ward to ward and doctor to doctor a firm system was introduced whereby each patient was made the continuing responsibility of a consultant psychiatrist whether in hospital or attending out-patient clinics. Severalls was divided into a psycho-geriatric unit and five other units.

Implementation of the firm system was completed by June 1963 with the appointment of a fifth consultant.

By 1964 Severalls Hospital had a catchment area of most of Essex and part of East Hertfordshire. The population at risk was 714,000. There were about 415 general practitioners, 13 mental welfare officers and 7 psychiatric social workers. The hospital is run on a unit (team or firm) system. Each unit is headed by a consultant assisted by two junior doctors, one social worker and a secretary. Five consultants, collectively, hold twenty-seven out-patient clinic sessions and make about twelve domiciliary visits per week. Emergency admissions are the responsibility of the consultant who is 'on call' for one week in rotation. Patients remain under the care of the same consultant in hospital or out-patients unless they or their general practitioner request a change. If a consultant makes a domiciliary visit on a patient already under the care of another consultant, he becomes responsible from then on for that patient.

Routinely, admissions or re-admissions are organised as follows:

(1) Patients seen in an out-patient clinic by a consultant or his junior are admitted directly to one of his beds in the admission villa common to all units or into the two wards and two villas allocated to him in the hospital.

(2) If patients are unable to attend the out-patient clinic, they can be seen on a domiciliary visit.

(3) Emergency admissions are arranged either after a visit by a consultant, or, if that is not possible because of hospital commitments, distance, fog, etc., after consultation over the telephone. A letter from the general practitioner giving details of the symptoms, their duration, evolution and response to treatment together with relevant information about family quarrels and socio-domestic-economic factors is expected.

(4) Psycho-geriatric emergency admissions are admitted to the consultant's own beds and take their turn on the waiting list for admission to the psycho-geriatric unit. A comprehensive psycho-geriatric service (Whitehead, 1965; Barton, 1966) with 324 beds provides a month-in, month-out service, a day hospital with 100 places and accepts patients on a waiting list. Priorities for admission are reviewed daily. The service tries to enable general practitioners to relieve families and patients with senile dementia by sharing problems of nursing and supervision early on in the illness, thus preventing precipitate admission and extending the families' tolerance for the remainder of the patient's life.

Each unit consists of two first-storey wards in the main hospital building (one for women and one for men) and two villas. There is a suite of four offices between each unit's wards in the main building. One office is shared by the consultant with his junior doctors. A second is for the unit secretary, a third for the unit social worker and the fourth is shared by the assistant matron and assistant chief male nurse attached to each firm.

There is an admission unit for new patients and each consultant has ten beds for women and seven for men. The majority of patients admitted to Severalls have been treated in this unit since 1960.

Prompt treatment allows early discharge before the patient's niche in the community is lost through accommodation being sold or tenancy terminated or marital infidelity of partners.

One of the problems of psychiatric hospitals is the constantly changing population of junior doctors, some of whom are of inferior training and personal calibre, and often with no psychiatric experience.

To counter this, each firm has an assistant matron and assistant chief male nurse who transmit the policies of the consultant and hospital to nursing staff. The assistant matron is responsible for backing up the ward sister, for arranging group discussions with nurses, for ensuring the wards maintain a therapeutic programme and that each patient is regularly scrutinised as to whether she is capable of achieving more than at present and whether the quality of her life is the best possible that can be obtained. Representations to the matron, the physician superintendent or directly to the hospital secretary for equipment, furnishings, redecoration or modifications of organisation are part of the assistant matrons' obligation and commitment.

Theoretically this should relieve medical staff of much administrative work and leave them free to carry out clinical psychiatry. In practice assistant matrons have changed frequently and newcomers do not take in the purpose of their appointment and nature of their role. Some doctors fail to appreciate the importance of their role and occupy their time and energy in other directions.

The most useful medical staff have been industrious, intelligent junior staff with a good basic knowledge of psychiatry who concentrate their efforts on individual patients without wasting time in therapeutic floundering, and who have appreciated the possibilities of the new organisation of Severalls and have learned to use it.

The background of reorganisation is shown in the physician superintendent's monthly reports to the H.M.C. and in his own diaries and correspondence, extracts from which are printed as Appendix 3.1 below.

NETHERNE HOSPITAL

by R. K. Freudenberg, M.D., D.P.M.

Netherne Hospital was opened in 1909. It is situated in the south-western fringe of Greater London and is responsible for psychiatric hospital and specialist services for adults. It serves three different local health authority areas with a total population of 535,295 in 1967. In 1909 it had twenty-three wards or villas (thirteen for women and ten for men). All these were closed except for two villas, one for each sex, where trusted and co-operative patients resided. This situation remained unchanged until the open-door policy began in 1942. Ten of the women's wards were in the north wing of the hospital, and eight of those for men in the west wing, leading off a halfmoon-shaped corridor. During this period the corridor was subdivided, before any ward could be entered, by glass partitions. This part of the hospital was generally, and is often still now, referred to as the main building.

A closed admission unit, one wing for men and another for women, was provided in a separate building. Another closed and separate building was used for subnormal women patients. The total number of beds available in 1909 was 960.

During the period from 1909 to about 1942 discipline was strict for both staff and patients. Each unit was surrounded by railings. The male and female staff were not allowed to talk to each other while on duty. Many slept in small rooms attached to the wards. The men had to obtain permission from the medical superintendent to marry, and the behaviour of staff and patients was controlled by a book of rules and regulations which tended to expand yearly. An elaborate formal and informal system of punishments and rewards existed to control the patients' behaviour. The medical staff during their rounds could not talk to patients individually, but were always accompanied by either matron or chief male nurse or one of their assistants and the sister or charge nurse of the ward. Older nurses report that enquiries were first addressed to the more senior nurse, who would in turn ask the charge nurse, who would reply to the senior nurse, who would then duly reply to the doctor. All wards and villas were staffed both during the day and night. All patients were detained compulsorily until 1932 when the Mental Treatment Act introduced the voluntary patient, but the majority of patients remained in hospital under compulsion until a more liberal policy started in the early 1940s. The main emphasis was placed on personal hygiene and physical health.

During the period 1909 to 1942 patients were employed in the utility departments of the hospital, on ward domestic work and on the farm, but occupational opportunities only existed for about 100–200 patients. The majority had to pass the day in idleness or often in useless occupations like polishing dustbins or ward buckets, apart from the brass doorhandles, etc. They were deprived of their possessions, and wore hospital clothing. Communications with their relations or the community were severely restricted.

Admission rates were less than one-third of the present numbers. The only community services for the mentally ill were emergency services for the compulsory removal of patients to hospital on magistrates' orders by so-called duly authorised officers employed by local health authorities.

In 1932 a new unit of 120 beds for elderly patients was added to the hospital, with two wards for each sex, and seven additional villas, three for men and four for women. This increased the total number of available beds to 1,480. In 1939 an annexe was acquired in a nearby village with 300 beds, raising the total number of beds to 1,620. The main development since the opening of the hospital was an increase in the number of beds, as it was thought during this period that this was in the best interests of the patients. In 1948 it provided a total of 1,918 beds. In 1965 the population served remained around 610,580, but the number of beds had reduced to 1,718 and in 1967 to 1,640. On 31 December 1968 the population served had reduced to 536,995 and the beds to 1,557.

The gradual reduction of beds used was not a planned procedure, but probably happened for a number of reasons, partly the development of alternative facilities, partly changing attitudes and policies of management of institutions such as psychiatric hospitals, and to alterations in the size of the population served.

Though development proceeded in three main areas, the order of priority was dictated by a combination of local circumstances and personal preferences. In this context I shall not discuss psycho-geriatric services in detail, as the comparative study was concerned with patients of working age. The first area of development was the creation of out-patient facilities in the early thirties, which have increased dramatically since 1945. Almost daily, diagnostic treatment and follow-up clinics are now held in all the four district general hospitals in the population area served. At these clinics initially hospital-based social-work staff attended (1946), but local authority or community-based social workers are becoming increasingly involved.

In 1966 the majority of patients were seen at such clinics before admission and 64 per cent of all discharged patients were followed up there. The re-admission rate was 46 per cent. With the expansion of out-patient services early treatment in-patient facilities were improved. Initially (1945–1951) the hospital social service department was mainly concerned with admission, and out-patients. Now it employs seven social workers, four of them qualified psychiatric social workers, one student and two unqualified workers with nursing and practical social work experience. The department co-operates closely with twenty community social workers at present employed by the three local health authorities served by the hospital.

The second area began to be tackled in 1952 and was concerned with the social environment provided for hospital in-patients, particularly those of working age whose stay in hospital remained prolonged. Emphasis was placed on basic needs like privacy and individual possessions, stimulating daily activities, etc. This development was associated with the realisation that early treatment only produced limited results, as only a minority of the patients left the hospital symptom-free.

Local circumstances at that time were not favourable to a more rapid development of community-based facilities, partly because of the multiplicity of local authorities in the area served by the hospital and partly because of negative attitudes towards such development. The obstacles to this kind of development still remain considerable. This phase therefore concentrated on the whole range of social circumstances, which could hinder or help a patient's progress in hospital, and on better preparation for discharge by providing a wide range of social and work activities.

The third phase, beginning in about 1960 and still in progress now, is concerned with the development of various alternatives to in-patient provision, such as day hospital facilities nearer to the population served by the hospital, the provision of alternative residential accommodation in the form of hostels, supervised lodgings, etc., a range of workshop facilities in the community, and generally closer integration and improvement in communications between the facilities provided by the hospital service and that of local authorities.

GENERAL ORGANISATION OF IN-PATIENT FACILITIES FOR
SHORT- AND LONG-STAY IN-PATIENTS

The hospital wards have for some time been divided between four medical teams. Each has a short-stay mixed admission unit for both sexes for younger, middle-aged and elderly patients, suffering from functional disorders. These units are related to certain geographical areas and have their out-patient departments in the district general hospitals situated in this area. Each team also relates to the local authority mental health services of their respective areas and has regular meetings, case and review conferences, at the out-patient department, at the local authority's premises, the day hospital or the respective in-patient unit. These acute short-stay units and their primary catchment areas are only concerned with a part of the total population area served by the hospital, and overlap with the secondary catchment areas, covering the whole population areas served by the hospital, and with the more specialised teams for psychiatrically handicapped patients of working age and their rehabilitation, and for psycho-geriatric patients and their short-stay treatment, rehabilitation and prolonged care units.

Two of the medical teams, with one consultant each and 1½ junior staff each, have 30 in-patient beds and their respective out-patient and other community responsibilities, and if necessary refer rehabilitation and psycho-geriatric problems to the more specialised teams. The other two teams therefore have additional responsibilities in relation to the total population area served. One is, apart from the short-stay unit, concerned with all psycho-geriatric wards and is responsible for the waiting list of psycho-geriatric patients and the preventive and after-care services for such patients, in collaboration with local authority social work staff, for the total catchment area of the hospital, assisted by three more junior medical staff.

Another is divided into two sections under one consultant and two juniors in each and, apart from a short-stay treatment unit, is concerned with all longer-term patients of working age to whom rehabilitation services particularly apply. This team is also responsible for all workshops, the staff involved in these and the general policy for rehabilitation facilities, both inside and outside hospital, supported by a rehabilitation committee, of which the principal nursing officer, the head occupational therapist, the recreation officer, the senior psychiatric social worker, the supervisor of the employment office, the industrial officer, the disablement resettlement officer, and the heads of the local authorities' mental health departments are members. A patients payments committee of the same composition regularly discusses principles of payments to patients, policy changes, etc. with the finance officer of the Group.

This distribution of the in-patient units developed mainly because of the special interests of members of the medical staff, and therefore their preference for and greater competence in dealing with certain patients. It was also considered that two small short-stay units, with no additional in-patient responsibilities for the medical staff, would offer better opportunities for junior medical staff in the early stages of their training. The short-stay unit attached to the rehabilitation team also serves as a re-admission and treatment unit for rehabilitation patients who have relapsed and may be in need of short-term intensive treatment. No increase in medical staffing can be expected in the foreseeable future.

ORGANISATION OF IN-PATIENT FACILITIES FOR THE
REHABILITATION OF DISABLED PATIENTS

(a) Living area

Clinical and work assessment of each patient led to a classification of the wards for long-staying patients of working age according to the degree of their primary disability from the most severe to the mildest. Wherever the physical structure of a building allowed it, mixed wards were established, with joint day accommodation for both sexes. Otherwise, what used to be the male and female sides of the hospital were changed in so far as wards for men or wards for women alternate as far as the preponderance of 2:1 women to men in the hospital makes this possible. A classification of wards according to degree of disability made it easier to tailor programmes to a particular disability. In wards for the most severely disabled, programmes were more structured, with a daily schedule of activities starting from getting-up time in the morning at 7 a.m. to bedtime. All such daily schedules were discussed at staff and patient meetings. More severely disabled patients also needed a higher nurse–patient ratio (i.e. one nurse to ten patients on wards for the most severely disabled, and night observation). This ratio decreases as disabilities become milder. At the top of the ladder as far as living is concerned are reasonably well-motivated patients who need least support and are all in paid employment, where one nurse is concerned with 130 patients, and there are no night staff.

(b) *Work area*

One of the principles we arrived at for work rehabilitation programmes, which have developed since 1956, was the provision of paid work opportunities for all disabled patients down to the severest degrees of disability.

The paid work facilities incorporate all the employment opportunities provided by the maintenance and utility services of the hospital, the laundry and domestic work as well as industrial sub-contract work and offices for clerical work. Regular work assessments are made and payments are adjusted to output, with a bonus and fine system in relation to good or bad attendance. They are co-ordinated into graded work situations, of which there are by now about 100. Before work placement, disabilities, assets and inclinations of patients are taken into account, to which the degree of support and supervision required is adjusted. The more severely disabled patients requiring a high supervisor–worker ratio, i.e. 1:8 or 10, gradually decreasing to the least disabled where it is nearer to what applies in industry outside.

Generally, paid industrial work tends to be used for the more disabled and those needing special assessment and preparation for resettlement. Maintenance or utility work, where there is least supervision, is given to those who have maintained or developed good work habits and have become self motivated. 'Avocational work' is used for those who are not disabled, but ill.

In many instances people have concerned themselves mainly with creating work programmes simply by creaming off the least disabled patients in the hospital or in the community. We have set out to create rehabilitation facilities and paid work programmes for all, even the most disabled in all age groups, because we believed that only then could a real change in the function of the services from custody to rehabilitation occur (see Tables 3.1–3.3, pp. 196–8).

No placements in work outside hospital are made for disabled patients without adequate trial in work situations in the hospital. There are limitations to hospital-based workshops and full use is made therefore of the opportunities provided or supported by the Ministry of Labour, such as industrial rehabilitation units, government training centres, industrial therapy organisations, or sheltered industries for the disabled provided by local authorities or voluntary organisations for bridging the gap between hospital and open employment.

THE FUNCTION OF THE MULTI-DISCIPLINARY TEAM IN RELATION TO REHABILITATION

Since the development of comprehensive rehabilitation programmes, regular assessment meetings were introduced, which are now held in all units. At these the psychiatrist reports on the clinical condition of the patient, the nursing staff on the general social behaviour on the ward, the occupational therapist or work supervisor on work performance. A rehabilitation programme tailored to individual needs is then formulated for each patient. Such meetings are mainly held during the lunch break.

EMPLOYMENT OFFICE

A central office was created in 1961, where every patient in the hospital is reported on admission, transfer or discharge. This office keeps a personal card, showing each individual patient allocated to the particular work he is doing. It also calculates the patient's pay, keeps records of payments received by patients from other sources, and copies of work reports which are taken to assessment meetings. It is therefore continuously in touch with the patient's work situation and files objective records of the type of work and the patient's work performance (Ekdawi *et al.*, 1968).

In the third phase of development, the community-based facilities expanded, which has led as far as rehabilitation facilities are concerned to:

(*a*) day patients working in hospital-based workshops, i.e. at present 34;

(*b*) day patients attending a separate day hospital, with up to 50 places, with an industrial workshop;

(*c*) after-care services for resettled workers: (i) workers' meeting in the evenings, attended by groups of up to 50 patients; (ii) evening clinics;

(*d*) the creation of a separate day hospital at Netherne with 50–60 places and separate industrial workshop facilities.

Attendances at out-patient clinics in general hospitals and at day hospitals amounted to about 80,000 at 31 December 1968.

Alternative residential accommodation is provided in five hostels in which the local authorities so far have about 100 places, otherwise patients are placed in 'digs' if their social competence makes this possible.

PROBLEMS AND CHANGES IN THE REHABILITATION SERVICES

The industrial workshop facilities and other work opportunities at the hospital or in the community can now offer paid work for those disabled patients who contact our services. In 1965 309 were unoccupied and in 1968 369; these consisted mainly of elderly and infirm patients and of new admissions. On 31 December 1962 801 patients were aged 60+. On 31 December 1968 this figure had declined to 788. The number of patients with duration of stay of more than two years aged under 60 decreased from 574 on 13 November 1962 to 559 on 3 November 1964 and to 444 on 2 February 1969. This figure could be reduced further if more sheltered work and living facilities were available in the community. Occupied industrial workshop places in the hospital similarly declined from 410 in 1962 to 271 in 1968, but patients working outside hospital increased in number from 79 on 31 December 1962 to 104 on 31 December 1964, and reduced to 102 on 13 December 1968. One of the problems that have occurred is that it is becoming increasingly difficult to find stabilised working patients for admission to the resettlement unit of the hospital, and the criteria for admission to it have changed in various respects. Originally only patients of working age with a duration of stay of over two years were admitted. Now the criteria are a duration of illness of two years+. Originally 135 beds were available in this unit. It cannot now be filled and the unit is about to be reduced to 70 beds, 35 for patients working outside and 35 working in hospital. This is hostel-type accommodation with one nursing staff and no night staff.

Another reason for the reduction of patients suitable for this type of facility is the increasing age of the patient population. Hostel-type accommodation for patients aged 60+ has increased and is now available for 108 men and 156 women.

Various changes had to be made in workshops. Workshop places for 'sheltered work' for older age groups had to be increased.

The overall organisation and staffing of the industrial departments has changed in so far as the industrial officer and industrial supervisors under him are responsible for the supply of industrial work, work process, layout, stores, etc., and occupational therapists for assessment, placing and movement of patients in consultation with the supervisor and medical staff. This seems to ensure greater stability and the development of industrial methods. The determining factor is more to ensure a layout best suited from an industrial point of view, which generally provides work opportunities of varying complexity, and to fit in patients accordingly rather than to have working groups of severely disabled together, which was the practice in the early days.

DEFINITION OF REHABILITATION STAGES

Rehabilitation Stage 1: Most severely disabled in structured work and living situation. Generally not in mixed units. 1:10 day staff, 1 night staff. More supervision at work 1:8, also training wage, often on indigent moneys. No self-motivation. Not suitable for utility work. Mostly on basic industrial subcontract work.

Rehabilitation Stage 2: Severely disabled. Generally in mixed units. Still needing highly structured programme both for work and living area. Not stabilised. Not yet self-motivated. Training wage up to lower piece-rate earning. Not suitable for utility work. Mostly on basic industrial subcontract work. In need of night supervision.

Rehabilitation Stage 3: Moderate–severe disabilities. More stabilised. Somewhat more self-motivated. Still fairly structured work programme, mostly industrial subcontract work. Lower piece-rate workers. No utility workers. Not in need of night supervision.

Rehabilitation Stage 4: Pre-resettlement. Patients are stabilised. Work in higher grade industrial subcontract or utility work. Reasonably self-motivated. Some working outside hospital. Not in need of night supervision. Handicaps slight–moderate.

Rehabilitation Stage 5: Resettlement. Patients are stabilised, work in higher grade industrial subcontract or utility work. Better self-motivation than Stage 4. Handicaps slight. Placement in open or sheltered work in the community. Approaching point of economic independence.

CHANGES INTRODUCED DURING 1960–1964

In 1961 both the physician superintendent (R. K. Freudenberg) and one of the consultants (D. H. Bennett), particularly interested in rehabilitation, left the services of the hospital for employment elsewhere. Shortly afterwards the matron of the hospital died and the secretary retired. A prolonged period of temporary acting appointments followed until the hospital became part of a general hospital group in 1964. Late in 1964 the physician superintendent returned to his previous appointment at Netherne.

As the number of patients working outside hospital, while remaining resident, increased considerably in the years from 1960 to 1964, it became necessary to hold doctors' meetings outside working hours. At these meetings difficulties at work or other personal problems are discussed and individual interviews arranged if required. Such meetings started in 1962 and have been held regularly since at the hospital and also for discharged day hospital patients at the day hospital.

Case review meetings were expanded in 1962 and were held for about two hours each week at Downs House and Pendellswood. One-hour staff and case-review meetings were held at Broadwood, Figgswood and Harpswood weekly, and one more detailed case conference weekly. Monthly staff meetings were started for Figgswood, Broadwood, Harpswood, Pendellswood and Downs House. A number of different social clubs for the patients of working age have developed since 1963. One functions at Downs House for both Downs House and Pendellswood patients. Another was established for Broadwood, Figgswood and Harpswood—the Villas Club, a third for Elizabeth and Gainsborough Wards, and a fourth for Clive and Disraeli Wards.

These clubs organised programmes for leisure activities, outside working hours, now with the help of one especially appointed recreation officer.

Admission to the resettlement unit is now not confined to patients who have been in hospital for more than two years but includes an increasing number of disabled patients who have been ill for more than two years but had remained in the community.

Changes in the occupational facilities 1960–1964

Since the completion of one workshop (The Vale) called the rehabilitation workshop for patients reaching the resettlement stage, which was opened in 1956, another workshop was built and opened in 1959 (Downs View). The latter was originally used for severely disabled patients.

In 1960, the occupational therapy department still had separate heads, one for men and the other for women, though both sexes worked in each of the departments. The industrial subcontracts expanded during the year and by the end of 1962 410 patients were working on industrial subcontract work in three workshops, Downs View, The Vale and Woodcote. One of the workshops, Downs View, catered for severely disabled patients and the other, The Vale, provided higher grade work for the more moderately handicapped, while Woodcote catered for the middle-aged to elderly. An industrial officer was appointed in 1961. In 1962 a part-time van driver and a van were acquired for the industrial departments. In 1963 the chief male occupational therapist retired and in 1964 a head occupational therapist was appointed for the whole hospital.

The wards remained the same during the period 1960–1964 except for the reduction in the number of patients in the closed ward for women to twenty-four and the transfer of this ward to a structurally smaller unit.

CONCLUSIONS

A short account of the development of hospital and community-based facilities was given, with particular reference to patients of working age in need of rehabilitation. A graded system of living and work areas has been developed, which is moving away from a strict classification in streams to more comprehensive work units dictated by industrial needs. In both living and work areas greater provision is being made for sheltered living and work situations such as hostel-type accommodation and 'sheltered workshops'. Difficulties resulting from existing staff shortages are reduced by a system of review by the multi-disciplinary team and other organisation innovations such as the employment office. A special system of payment for work related for performance, with bonus and fines systems, and a basic training wage in the early stages has improved attendance and work performance.

APPENDIX 3.1

Diary of Change at Severalls Hospital

by Russell Barton, M.B., M.R.C.P., D.P.M.

1960

1 Jan. New Physician Superintendent took office. Discussions with medical, nursing and administrative staff on the aims, methods and roles in a psychiatric service.

7 Jan. Programme of open wards and 'decertification' started.

13 Jan. Nursing Education Committee formed. Discussions on combating illness, O.T., industrial therapy started.

18 Jan. Doctors elected mess president and secretary.

19 Jan. Disablement resettlement officer begins weekly visits.

20 Jan. 'Forum meetings' for medical staff, ward sisters, charge nurses and other nursing staff started.

25 Jan. Out-patient clinics at Colchester increased to 4 sessions weekly. Copies of *Institutional Neurosis* distributed to every ward.

27 Jan. Course of public lectures by physician superintendent started (about 1 every 2 weeks to local societies).

1 Feb. Cement and concrete team making blocks, paving slabs and kerb-stones begins with 6 patients.

3 Feb. Patient's contact with the outside world stressed. Discussions with medical and nursing staff opened.

10 Feb. Control of Infection Committee started.

12 Feb. Concept of patients' 'territory' stressed to nursing staff. Patients' need for personal possessions, friends and events discussed.

14 Feb. Unrestricted Visiting declared. (From 9.00 a.m. to 9.00 p.m.)

19 Feb. Discussions on patients' clothing started.

22 Feb. New combined wardrobe, ward divider, chest of drawers, bookshelf mocked up. 9″ width per bed allows all these facilities. Discussions with nurses on hairdressing and improvement of personal appearance of patients started.

25 Feb. Plans for factory finalised—a Dutch Barn and window frames to be purchased by end of financial year. Walls to be of breezeblocks made in hospital.

1 March. Dr J. K. Wing and Mr G. Brown from M.R.C. unit arrive.

3 March. Deteriorated patients begin scraping and painting rooms in a ward bombed 17 years previously.

18 March. Course of 40 lectures for medical staff and general practitioners in neurology, neuro-anatomy and psychiatry started. Average 25 doctors attend.

31 March. Communications system of distributing information circulars developed: (*a*) doctors, (*b*) doctors and senior nursing staff, (*c*) doctors and all nursing staff, (*d*) all staff.

7 April. Programme of patients cooking cakes and light meals on wards begun. Cookers to be fitted in more ward kitchens.

14 April. Aims and objects of industrial therapy report by Dr Barton. Weekly meetings of industrial therapy staff to discuss policy and organisation started.

20 April. Now 19 men and 6 women patients working outside hospital.

21 April. Approval and assurances of co-operation with industrial therapy objectives received from Colchester Chamber of Commerce and trades council.

25–27 April. Refresher course for postgraduate nurses organised at Severalls. Nursing staff of other hospitals attend. Theme is institutional neurosis—its cause and cure.

2 May. Drive started to get all friendless patients a card and gift at birthdays and Christmas. Voluntary workers encouraged.

10 May. Nursing staff visit Cheadle Royal to see the industrial therapy developed there.

14 May. Conference of Chief Male Nurses.

18 May. Discussions on abuses of drugs with nursing staff.

23 May. Beauty Salon opened and nurse sent to Atkinson beauty salon for course in beauty preparations and treatment.

6 June. Maternity unit moved to Severalls until 21 June. 17 babies born in Severalls.

10 June. All ground floor wards in main building (except A and B) converted to Psycho-geriatric Unit. Month in month out policy started. Elderly senile patients combed out of other wards.

11 July. Nursing staff start visiting homes of patients.

21 July. Maternity unit moved in and stayed until 23 August. 37 babies born.

29 July. Medical staff moved to new residence in former medical superintendent's house.

10 Aug. New clinical record introduced:—foolscap and continuous for I.P. and O.P. notes.

16 Aug. New admission procedure introduced. Patients now admitted directly to admission ward or geriatric unit.

17 Aug. Need for 1 extra consultant and 9 junior staff accepted by H.M.C.

30 Aug. 'Forum meetings' discontinued. (It had deteriorated from a group discussing aims and objects to a hostile group electing officers, keeping minutes and stirred up by one or two malcontents.)

24 Sept. Conference of Magistrates and Probation Officers.

26 Sept. Men's Industrial Therapy building finished.

30 Sept. Last patients taken off certificate. 15 (1 per cent) of patients were to remain certified. Chief Pharmacist retires.

10 Oct. Plans for Psychiatric Unit at Herts and Essex Hospital approved.

12 Oct. General Practitioners' informal discussion on the use of Severalls.

18 Oct. N.E.R.H.B. Psychiatric Advisory Committee Annual Dinner at Severalls.

24–26 Oct. Three-day Refresher Course for postgraduate nurses.

26 Oct. Last of boundary railings removed.

1 Nov. One-fifth of non-geriatric patients allocated at random to Dr Smith and one-fifth to Dr Calder (consultants).

16 Nov. Arrangements for geriatric patients to attend old people's clubs in Colchester.

29 Nov. N.E. Essex Branch of B.M.A.—Clinical evening.

30 Nov. Mental Welfare Officers, Medical and Nursing Staff meeting to discuss new Mental Health Act.

1 Dec. Myland Court (hitherto semi-private patients' unit) becomes admission unit. Each consultant to have 10 women's and 7 men's beds. Men and women patients to eat together—but this objective obstructed by staff who arrange two shifts, one men and women later.

16 Dec. Number of people being nursed in bed down to 5 (none hand fed).

21 Dec. Mayor opens Men's Psycho-geriatric Unit headquarters and 'month in—month out' policy publicly declared. Anglia TV appearance and discussion.

1961

2 Jan. Psychiatric out-patient clinics at Essex County Hospital increased to 9 sessions per week.

16 Jan. Departments of Electro-encephalography and Psychology given new quarters in former doctors' mess.

17 Jan. Course of 4 lectures in psychiatry, psychology, neurology and neuro-anatomy started and attended by hospital doctors, G.P.s, R.A.M.C. doctors.

6 Feb. Assistant Chief Male Nurse appointed from outside hospital staff. Regional Board approached for £1,000 per year for education in psychiatry for Severalls medical staff.

13 Feb. Only one men's and one women's ward remain locked.

22 Feb. Psychiatry Advisory Committee 'could not see their way clear to advise Board to pay for psychiatric training scheme' and advised R.H.B. against making financial provision for research at Severalls.

24 Feb. Talks on community care of discharged patients started in nurses and medical staff groups.

1 March. Regular ward meetings between nursing and medical staff encouraged on all wards. Mass clinical demonstrations attended by nurses and doctors discontinued.

27–29 March. Nurses' postgraduate refresher course. Community care and geriatric problems discussed.

30 March. Course of lectures completed. Average attendance 30 doctors.

19 April. Requirement for mental welfare officers to have permanent office in Severalls postponed by H.M.C. Statement of time and price taken to travel by public transport from Harlow and Canvey Island to Severalls— about 14s. and 4 hours—presented to H.M.C.

12 May. Day Hospital officially opened by M.O.H. for Colchester.

16 May. Clinical meeting attended by some 40 G.P.s.

18 May. One day course for newly ordained clergy held at Severalls Hospital. (This extended to 2 days has been held annually.)

19 May. Principle of consultant having right to admit to his own beds only and being committed to his patient in or out of hospital accepted at meeting with S.A.M.O. at Warley.

1 July. Twenty-four patients from Hill End Hospital spent two weeks at Severalls and a similar number of Severalls patients went to St Albans.

14 July. Plans for Women's Industrial Unit drawn up. Household management unit with 4 electric and 4 gas cookers, eight sinks and a dining-room started.

17 July. Occupational therapy extended into wards.

30 Sept. Clacton and District Trades Council visit Severalls.

9–11 Oct. Nurses' postgraduate refresher course held.

18 Oct. Chelmsford Trades University and Employers visit Severalls.

20 Oct. Reported that 16 men from men's psycho-geriatric unit had had holidays—10 had not slept out of Severalls for 20 to 48 years.

1 Nov. Plans for decoration of institutional corridors so that colour provides subliminal visual cues to destination approved (circular dated 26 October 1961).
30 Nov. Dr Rosenthal takes over his unit of two wards and 2 villas and one-fifth of non-geriatric patients.

1 Dec. Arrangements made for male staff nurse Jones and O.T. Mrs Jones to spend a week at Industrial Therapy projects at Bristol, Cheadle Royal and Netherne Hospitals and to make reports and proposals for new Women's Industrial Unit being erected.

1962

1 Jan. Regular Friday case conference instituted for medical staff.
16 Jan. Course of 40 lectures in psychiatry, neurology, neuro-anatomy and psychology for medical staff started (4 lectures weekly for 10 weeks).
29 Jan. Mayor of Colchester called a public meeting to form Friends of Severalls.

1 Feb. Application to S.A.M.O. for financial assistance for postgraduate education in psychiatry (letter).
20 Feb. 1st Committee meeting of Friends of Severalls.

26–28 March. Postgraduate refresher course for nurses held.

3 April. Dr L. C. Hurst appointed senior registrar.
11 April. Eight ladies and 4 men went to holidays in Clacton and 4 ladies and 8 men to a mental after-care hostel in Westcliff-on-Sea.
19 April. Mayor of Colchester opens Severalls medical library.

21 May. K ward, Dr Rosenthal's unit, now redecorated and divided into two wards.

1 June. Minister of Health opens hospital laundry.

3 July. Dr L. C. Hurst takes up duties as senior registrar.
7 July. Party of health visitors spend day at Severalls.
16 July. Dr W. K. Marshall, S.H.M.O. transferred to psycho-geriatric unit.

1 Aug. Psychiatric Unit at Herts and Essex Hospital, Bishops Stortford, opened. Dr J. A. Whitehead transferred from Severalls to Bishops Stortford for one year.
2 Aug. 3 medical students, one Yugoslavian, one Spanish and one Greek, spend 1 month at Severalls.
31 Aug. Mr Glen, senior psychologist, leaves.

3 Sept. Women's Industrial Unit completed. Places for 70 women available.

5 Sept. Dr Sidney Propert, M.D., F.R.C.P., Consultant Physician to Essex County Hospital, starts regular once-monthly visits to Severalls.

11 Sept. Course of 60 lectures (4 weekly) for medical staff started.

8 Oct. Catchment area of Severalls modified. Dagenham (population 115,000) lost but East Hertfordshire (population 133,000) gained. Discussions about surgical unit at Severalls started.

12 Oct. Conifer Close Hostel to be run by Essex County Council opened on Greenstead Estate.

18 Oct. Art Gallery and Picture Library opened by John Nash, R.A.

26 Oct. New front entrance brought into use.

29 Nov. Secretary of R.H.B. writes suggesting 'surplus accommodation at Severalls be utilised for general hospital purposes' and this would be facilitated by merger of H.M.C.s.

30 Nov. E.C.T. Unit at Myland Court completed.

1963

3 Jan. Course of lectures for medical staff at Severalls cancelled. A course at Herts and Essex Hospital to be given instead.

16 Jan. Out-patient sessions at Essex County increased to 8 per week, Chelmsford to 4 per week, Braintree to 2 per week and Clacton to 2 per week.

31 Jan. 6 male patients—the first batch of 50 men and 50 women—admitted from another hospital. These patients were very deteriorated, some with physical abnormalities and some incontinent of urine. Nursing staff openly hostile that Severalls should have to 'do another hospital's dirty work'.

7 Feb. Course of 10 lectures—once weekly demonstrations on psychiatry at Herts and Essex Hospital, Bishops Stortford—started by physician superintendent.

1 March. Work started on Castle Ward and Tamarisk Villa to accommodate Runwell patients who are repressed to be absorbed into units.

18 March. Dr Richard Fox appointed consultant. Additional J.H.M.O. added to the establishment making total establishment of 18 doctors.

21–23 April. Three-day postgraduate refresher couse for nurses held.

21 May. Talk with Mid-Essex division of B.M.A. on Severalls psychiatric service. S.A.M.O. in attendance. Dissastisfaction with admission process expressed. Need for improved communication system at Severalls (Personal call system and P.A.B.X.) discussed. Also need for an enquiry centre manned by a trained receptionist noted.

25 May. Friends of Severalls Fete. Over 5,000 people attended.
26–28 May. Open days. Over 1,000 members of public shown round hospital.

12 June. So far total of 48 patients transferred from another hospital—some mute, some incontinent, nearly all very regressed.
21 June. Discussion with visiting officers of Regional Board on communications—personal call system and use of telephones.
24 June. Dr Richard Fox started duties. Allocated 2 wards and two villas and one-fifth of non-geriatric patients.

1–5 July. Intensive one-week course in psychiatry for Essex County Council Health visitors organised. Lectures, case demonstrations, seminars and tutorials included.

1 Aug. Offices for consultants and their junior doctors in Myland Court completed.
31 Aug. Miss Robinson, Principal Tutor to Nurses Training School, retires owing to ill health.

13 Sept. Meeting of Essex County Council and officers of N.E.R.H.B. with physician superintendents at Romford to discuss provision of hostels for psychiatrically disordered people. Larger hostel at Stanway, already planned with consultation, nearing completion.
24–25 Sept. Two-day course in psychiatry for newly ordained clergy.

14 Oct. Dr J. A. Whitehead returns to Severalls as locum S.H.M.O. to run psycho-geriatric unit.
14–18 Oct. Repeat one-week course in psychiatry for health visitors.

7 Nov. Discussion of disablement resettlement officers in Phoenix Club.
20 Nov. H.M.C. formally approve establishment of O.P. clinics at Harwich, Halstead and Maldon.

1 Dec. Dr Whitehead, locum S.H.M.O., and Mr Adams, local authority P.S.W., develop scheme whereby elderly patients are fostered by families in the community.

1964

1 Jan. Dr Hurst resumes duties as senior registrar at Severalls.
4 Jan. Surgical unit officially opened by Mayor of Colchester. Consultant surgeon Mr Ronald Reid from Essex County Hospital. House surgeon to live in Severalls House.
31 Jan. Course of 10 weekly lectures and demonstrations by physician superintendent for medical staff from Severalls, other hospitals and general practitioners started.

17 Feb. Out-patient clinics now amounting to 24 sessions per week.

2–6 March. One-week repeat course of psychiatry for health visitors held.
18 March. Emergency domiciliary service for senile elderly patients living in the community proposed. Day hospital attendances at Severalls now 13. Proposals for improved transport to meet needs made.

3 April. Severalls Group Hospital Management Committee ceased to exist. Severalls now merged with Colchester Hospitals H.M.C. To become St Helena Group Hospital Management Committee.
20 April. Twenty-five day patients attending daily Monday to Friday.
24 April. Physician superintendent discusses with S.A.M.O. the principle of extending psychiatric services beyond hospital boundary. Also need for increase of establishment.
27 April. Dr J. K. Wing and Dr George Brown of Medical Research Unit visit Severalls for one week to re-assess remaining 82 patients of group of 100 which were selected at random and assessed in February 1960.

5 June. Principles and policy for traffic, car parks, sign-posting and directional aids to unit headquarters presented to H.M.C. Difficulty of recruitment of staff reported to H.M.C.
8 June. Mr L. G. R. Coombes appointed as Principal Nurse Tutor to Nurses Training School.

1–31 July. Two medical students—one from Rome and one from Germany —working at hospital.
13 July. Household Management Unit opened. Regressed and deteriorated patients groups emphasised.

20 Aug. Discussions with Nursing Officer of R.H.B. on nursing establishment held. Need for domestic workers stressed—many of the patients who did this work have been discharged. Patient peonage had many advantages—for the hospital.

1 Sept. Car washing unit added to Women's Industrial Unit.
9 Sept. Meeting with officers of local authority to discuss transport for day hospital. Physician superintendent predicts 100 patients will be attending day hospital by September 1965. (About 50 now attending daily.)
22–23 Sept. Two-day course in psychiatry for newly ordained clergy held at Severalls.

30 Oct. Mr Kniveton, Chief Male Nurse, retires.

17 Nov. Report on household management unit. 46 patients have attended. Shopping expeditions have proved successful and popular.

1965

1 Jan. Mr Corbett takes up duties as Chief Male Nurse. Two medical students from St Bartholomew's Hospital to attend for periods of 2 weeks as part of their curriculum from now on.

As a result of these changes, during the year 1965 there were 1,633 admissions to Severalls, 12,430 out-patient and domiciliary attendances at the various out-patient clinics and about 20,000 day hospital attendances.

At the psychiatric unit at Bishops Stortford there were 350 admissions, 2,000 out-patient attendances and 8,000 day hospital attendances.

4

THE NATURE OF INSTITUTIONALISM
IN MENTAL HOSPITALS

The material presented in this chapter extends and replicates the results of a previous study (Wing, 1961) in which it was shown that attitudes to discharge became more unfavourable, the longer the patient had been in hospital, independently of age and clinical condition. This gradual acquiescence in a state of life which precludes participation in the community outside hospital lies at the very heart of institutionalism.

In terms of the three interlocking theories presented in Chapter 1, it was expected that negative aspects of the clinical condition and social environment would be highly intercorrelated. Florid symptoms should be less in evidence if the environment were socially unstimulating and certainly not positively related to social poverty. The association between attitude to discharge and length of stay, independently of social and clinical condition (institutionalism), should be confirmed.

In order to examine the relationships between social, clinical and other relevant variables, two matrices of correlations were constructed, using fifteen of the main variables measured in 1960 and in 1964. Definitions of the variables have been given in Chapter 2. The matrices are presented in Tables 4.1 and 4.2 (pp. 199 and 200). It is evident from inspection that these are closely similar to each other although the measurements were made at an interval of four years and, in the case of the nurses' ratings and the inventories of personal possessions, by different people. Most of the subsequent discussion will be based on Table 4.1.

MEASURES OF THE SOCIAL ENVIRONMENT

The first five variables are measures of the social environment and the intercorrelations between them range in size from 0·43 to 0·70 ($p < 0.001$ in each case). That is, a patient who has little contact with the outside world is also likely to have few possessions, to spend much time doing nothing, and to be regarded pessimistically by the nurses. The common element in these five measurements may be called 'poverty of the social environment'. Each index, however, measures a different aspect of institutional life as experienced by the patients in the series and it would be unwise to submerge their separate identities and meanings into a single score. Since there were three quite different methods of measurement (nurses' questionnaire, sociologist's enquiry, and special inventory of possessions) the inter-correlations are unlikely to be spuriously high due to contamination.

CLINICAL CONDITION

Six indices of clinical condition are given in Tables 4.1 and 4.2. Three of them—social withdrawal score, flatness of affect and poverty of speech—are strongly related to each other. They might be labelled 'poverty of clinical condition'. The other three—incoherence of speech, coherently-expressed delusions and socially embarrassing behaviour—are less related to each other or to clinical poverty.

RELATIONSHIPS BETWEEN SOCIAL AND CLINICAL FACTORS

Social and clinical 'poverty' are strongly related together (coefficients ranging from 0·32 to 0·66) but 'florid' symptoms show a less consistent pattern (range of size 0·09–0·36). The strongest relationship is a negative one between favourable nurses' attitudes and socially embarrassing behaviour ($-0·36$). On the whole patients who talk coherently about delusions are less likely to show clinical poverty and also less likely to be living in conditions of environmental poverty.

Although ward restrictiveness cannot be included in the correlational analysis since it was not measured for all patients, Figure 4.3 (p. 201) is included to show that it is related to a clinical variable (social withdrawal) quite independently of another social factor (number of hours doing nothing). The interaction term is highly significant.

LENGTH OF STAY AND AGE

All the patients in the series had been in hospital at least two years in 1960. The mean length of stay was sixteen years. All the variables representing clinical and environmental poverty show small correlations with length of stay (size range 0·16 to 0·33). Attitude to

6

discharge is also related (0·39). The longer a patient has been in hospital, the more likely she is to experience socially impoverished conditions, the more likely to be socially withdrawn and to show poverty of affect and speech, and the more likely to be indifferent about leaving or actually to wish to stay. 'Florid' symptomatology is not related in this way; in fact, coherent delusions are expressed *less* often, the longer a patient has been in hospital.

Figure 4.4 (p. 202) shows the striking relationship between length of stay and three other factors, one 'primary' (social withdrawal), one 'secondary' (attitude to discharge), and one social (contact with the outside).

Age is related to length of stay, though not by as much as might have been expected (r = 0·45). The age and length of stay distribution of the patients are given in Chapter 5. Of 132 patients in the oldest age-group (51 to 60) less than half had been in hospital over twenty years, and about one-quarter had been resident ten years or less.

None of the five measures of poverty of social environment is correlated with age to an important extent (the correlations range from −0·16 to 0·05). Social withdrawal has a correlation of 0·03, and socially embarrassing behaviour score a correlation of 0·00 with age. It should be remembered that patients over 60 were not included in the series.

There is, however, a significant association between age and dose of phenothiazine (r = 0·21) indicating that older patients receive less medication. Phenothiazine is very little related to any other variable.

ATTITUDE TO DISCHARGE

Attitude to discharge was not rated on a scale, and correlation coefficients were calculated using two scores only (favourable and unfavourable). Moreover, patients who were mute or incoherent, who should properly be omitted since their attitudes are necessarily 'indifferent', have been included in order to give an overall impression of the interrelationships between variables. This means that there is an undue emphasis on correlations with measures of social and environmental poverty.

The marked tendency for attitudes to be less favourable the longer a patient has been in hospital is graphically illustrated in Figure 4.4.

The proportion of 99 per cent of short-stay (under two years) schizophrenic patients wanting to leave is taken from another study (Wing *et al.*, 1964). The data for the present series are presented in Table 4.5 (p. 203) in which the numbers of patients with various types of attitude, and the numbers excluded because of muteness or incoherence of speech, are shown within three length-of-stay groups. Omitting the mute and incoherent patients, there is a very highly significant relationship between the two variables ($\chi^2 = 37 \cdot 14$, df $= 6$, p $< 0 \cdot 001$, gamma $= 0 \cdot 45$).

Figure 4.6 (p. 203) shows the relationship between attitude to discharge and length of stay within two age groups. In patients under 45 years old, the association is significant, but not very strong ($\chi^2 = 5 \cdot 80$, df $= 1$, p $< 0 \cdot 02$). In patients aged 45–59, the association is very strong ($\chi^2 = 28 \cdot 85$, df $= 1$, p $< 0 \cdot 001$). On the other hand there is no significant relationship between attitude to discharge and age in either of the two length-of-stay groups.

Figure 4.7 (p. 204) shows graphically the relationship between attitude to discharge and length of stay when patients aged under and over 45 are examined separately. Two other variables, one social (degree of contact with the outside), the other clinical (social withdrawal and related behaviour), are controlled in the same way. In each case the two main variables remain strikingly associated.

Table 4.8 (p. 205) gives similar data, controlling in turn for three social variables (occupation score, favourable nurses' attitudes, and time doing nothing) and two clinical variables (flatness of affect and poverty of speech). In each case, there is a diminishing proportion of patients with favourable attitudes as length of stay increases, whether the controlling variable is high or low.

Finally, Table 4.9 (p. 205) shows the association between clinical category and attitude to discharge. Among those with moderate impairment only, 57 out of 97 (59 per cent) had some wish to leave. Among the 28 coherently-deluded patients rated, 23 (82 per cent) wanted to leave. Out of the remaining 85 patients rated, only 24 (28 per cent) had any wish for discharge.

PRE-ADMISSION FACTORS

Only 71 patients out of 273 (26 per cent) had ever been married. There is no relationship between marital status and length of stay or any of the other social and clinical variables.

The patients came from a wide range of social classes (classified according to father's occupation). The details are given in Chapter 5. There is no relationship, however, between class and length of stay or any of the social, clinical or attitudinal variables considered in this study.

Discussion

It is already clear that the 'end-state' in long-stay schizophrenic patients is not unitary. At least three different components can be detected which, although they affect each other, make an independent contribution to the final degree of impairment. These are, first, 'poverty of clinical condition'; secondly, florid symptomatology; and thirdly, unfavourable attitudes to discharge. 'Premorbid' factors, such as father's occupation, also play a part but only in selecting who is to become long-stay—not in affecting the actual degree of impairment. 'Clinical poverty' is a syndrome made up of the negative symptoms of schizophrenia—flatness of affect, poverty of speech and behaviour associated with social withdrawal. This is highly intercorrelated with 'poverty of the social environment' (lack of occupation, unfavourable nurses' attitudes, paucity of personal possessions, and lack of contact with the world outside).

One of our main hypotheses is thus confirmed, since the severity of primary impairments (in so far as they can be measured by negative symptoms) seems to be closely associated with degree of environmental under-stimulation. The direction of cause and effect is, however, crucial. Do withdrawn schizophrenic patients create their own social milieu, or does environmental poverty cause social withdrawal and allied symptoms? Much of the rest of this book will be devoted to trying to answer this question. The contribution of ward restrictiveness is also of interest since it seems to be associated with social withdrawal independently of other measures of environmental poverty.

The degree of withdrawal in many of the schizophrenic patients we interviewed is much greater than would be expected in any other group of people, such as the long-term inmates of internment camps or prisons, who have been exposed to a closed institution for long periods of time. Moreover, it is clear from other studies (e.g. Brown *et al.*, 1966) that negative symptoms are common in schizophrenic patients who have never stayed in hospital for more than a few months. We shall not, therefore, include 'clinical and social poverty' as a part of 'institutionalism'. This matter will be discussed again in Chapter 10, after the rest of the evidence has been presented.

The other type of primary impairment in schizophrenia is evidenced by the group of florid symptoms. Incoherence of speech and socially embarrassing behaviour are correlated with social factors to a much lower degree, but according to the same general pattern, as are negative symptoms. They are relatively uncommon, as would be expected according to the theory that over-stimulation exacerbates them. Coherently-expressed delusions, in contrast, stand out as having favourable implications on almost all counts. Patients with this symptom are less likely to show 'clinical poverty', less likely to be living in conditions of social under-stimulation, more likely to be short-stay, and more likely to wish to leave hospital (though their attitudes may be unrealistic). In terms of our hypotheses, they are resistant to the ill-effects of poverty of their social milieu compared to schizophrenic patients who have predominantly negative symptoms or incoherence of speech, who are vulnerable to these ill-effects.

So far as secondary impairments are concerned, our main measure was attitude to discharge, which represents a whole complex of secondary adaptations to the institutional environment (Wing, 1961). Table 4.9 (p. 205) shows that a primary impairment is also involved here; mute patients, for example, and those who are completely incoherent, do not have measurable attitudes, but, in terms of their behaviour, seem indifferent about leaving. Even when these patients are excluded, both severity and type of symptomatology are related to attitude to discharge. Thus we do not have a pure measure of a secondary impairment. Nevertheless, it is clear that attitude to discharge is related to length of stay, independently of other factors, such as age, type and severity of symptomatology or social surroundings (even degree of contact with the outside). This is what our hypothesis requires and it confirms previous findings in male patients (Wing, 1961; Freeman, Mandelbrote and Waldron, 1965).

The use of length of stay as a key variable requires comment. It is not permissible to infer temporal trends from cross-sectional data unless the effect of selection can be allowed for. The methodological problems have already been discussed in Chapter 1. However, the omission of patients who had been in hospital for less than two years makes it unlikely that the relationships between attitude to discharge and length of stay can be entirely accounted for in terms of the earlier discharge of patients who wanted to leave.

We shall use the term 'institutionalism' to describe this general relationship between length of stay in an institution, which both constrains an individual to stay for a long time and limits his contacts with the outside world, and the gradual adoption of an attitude of indifference to leaving. As we saw in Chapter 1, the literary evidence for such a relationship is very suggestive. A fundamental social law is presumably involved, which is as apparently trivial as Popper foresaw all social laws would turn out to be. The longer a person persists in one form of activity, or undergoes one form of experience, the more difficult it will be for him to choose any other and the less he will want to do so. This applies to such diverse social activities or statuses as occupation and nationality. It also applies to residence in institutions.

'Institutionalism' and 'clinical poverty' are not necessarily found together. Of the 97 patients with only a moderate degree of clinical impairment, 28 per cent wanted to leave, 31 per cent were ambivalent and 41 per cent had unfavourable attitudes (nearly all wanted to stay). The relationship to length of stay was very strong in this group of moderately-impaired patients. However, when the two factors do occur concurrently, so that the patient is both severely impaired because of negative symptoms and an impoverished social environment, *and* because of an unfavourable attitude to discharge, the potential for rehabilitation and chances for eventual resettlement outside must appear very poor. This is the typical picture presented by the patient in the 'back ward'. In such patients, the immediate problem is to reduce the primary disabilities, but even if successful, this will not necessarily affect the secondary impairments which need special measures of their own. These matters are analysed further in Chapters 6 and 7.

Summary

1. Five measures of the immediate social environment in which 273 long-stay schizophrenic women were living in 1960 formed a highly intercorrelated cluster: 'poverty of the social milieu'. A patient who had little contact with the outside world was also likely to own few personal possessions, to have little constructive occupation, to spend much time doing nothing and to be regarded pessimistically by ward nurses.

2. Three measures of clinical condition were also clearly related to each other—social withdrawal, flatness of affect, and poverty of speech. Patients who were living in the most under-stimulating social environment were likely to show the greatest clinical poverty, and this complex was likely to be more severe the longer the patient had been in hospital. Much of the rest of this book is devoted to analysing the direction of cause and effect.

3. Both environmental and clinical poverty were associated with unfavourable attitudes to discharge but, independently of these associations, attitudes to discharge became progressively more unfavourable with length of stay. This was not due to age or other intervening variables. It is suggested that there was a gradual process of attitude change, similar to that which might occur in any individual who remained in a closed institution for many years. This process was named 'institutionalism'.

4. Florid symptoms such as incoherence of speech, coherently-expressed delusions and socially embarrassing behaviour were relatively uncommon. Incoherence of speech showed a pattern of relationship to other variables which was closely similar to that of poverty of speech but less strong. Patients with coherent delusions were less likely to show 'clinical poverty', less likely to be living in conditions of social under-stimulation, more likely to be short-stay and more likely to wish to leave hospital.

5. Age seemed to be of little independent significance except that phenothiazines were less used as patients became older. Dose of phenothiazine was not related to any of the other variables. Marital status at the time of admission, and father's occupation, were not related to length of stay.

6. There was an important association between length of stay, age and unfavourable attitude to discharge, independently of social and clinical poverty, suggesting a gradual process of attitude change which might occur whenever an individual remained in one setting for many years.

5

DIFFERENCES BETWEEN
THE HOSPITALS IN 1960[1]

We assumed that there would be marked differences between the three hospitals in 1960, which the data concerning the total series of patients presented in Chapter 4 have obscured. The aims of the present chapter are, first, to describe the three social environments and, secondly, assuming that they do differ in important ways, to see whether there are equivalent clinical differences between the three groups of patients. We hypothesised that social poverty and clinical poverty should go together—but that, if anything, florid symptoms would be found in association with the most stimulating social conditions. Attitudes to discharge should be significantly related to length of stay at all three hospitals and there would be little difference between the three groups of patients in the proportion who wanted to leave.

AGE, LENGTH OF STAY AND OCCUPATION OF FATHERS

The composition of the three samples in respect of age and length of stay is set out in Tables 5.1 and 5.2 (p. 206).

The distributions are not significantly different at the three hospitals. However, since Mapperley tends to have more patients in the 51–60 age group, and more in the over-21-years length-of-stay group, it will be necessary to allow for this in the subsequent analysis.

The occupation of the patients' fathers was classified according to the system of Hall and Moser (1954), and differences between the three hospitals are shown in Table 5.3 (p. 207).

An effort was made to obtain this information by writing to the relatives of patients who could not give it themselves, but it was not available for 51 patients (19 per cent). There was considerable variation between hospitals ($\chi^2 = 29.54$, df = 8, p < 0.001). In particular, the fathers of patients at Netherne Hospital had significantly more often been engaged in professional or managerial occupations compared with either of the other two hospitals.

[1] Part of the material in this chapter has been presented in two earlier papers (Brown and Wing, 1962; Wing and Brown, 1961).

SOCIAL ENVIRONMENTS PROVIDED BY THE THREE HOSPITALS

Ward restrictiveness scores

Each patient in the three samples was given the score for his ward, and the sum of scores was divided by the number of patients in the sample. The mean scores are expressed as percentages of the possible total of 50. The average score for Netherne Hospital was 27 (range 8–62, eight wards studied). For Mapperley Hospital it was 40 (range 20–54, five wards studied), and for Severalls Hospital, 66 (range 11–89, eight wards studied). These mean scores represent the combined experience of the patients in the various samples.

Measures of amenities provided on these wards also showed large differences between the hospitals. For example, a count was made of all lockers (whatever their size), wardrobes, dressing tables and chests of drawers on each of the selected wards. In Netherne Hospital there were 522 such articles of furniture for 378 patients in the eight wards studied (1·4 per patient), in Mapperley Hospital 418 articles for 191 patients in five wards studied (2·9 each), and in Severalls Hospital 113 articles for 500 patients in eight wards (0·2 each).

A number of sisters and nurses at Mapperley and Severalls commented spontaneously in the course of the interview about the insufficiency of staff to deal properly with patients. There was only one spontaneous comment at Netherne. Typical remarks were: 'There is very little staffing. Patients are left alone three afternoons a week. They need someone to get them going—on things like a game of cards.' 'It is very, very difficult to deal with withdrawal—we've never enough time. I would like to get them more occupied, and more staff to take them for walks—to get them happily tired. They spend too much time sitting in the Day Room.' 'On a ward like this there is not much chance to draw them out—we've not enough staff.' 'We have to talk to them in the evenings if we can—there's never enough time during the day...we don't do justice to the lost ones.'

It is difficult to obtain a satisfactory comparative index of the ratio of nursing staff to patients because much time may be spent by patients away from the wards during the day. A special 1 in 4 sample of *all* female patients showed that at Netherne only 6 per cent remained during the day in the selected wards, 43 per cent at Mapperley, and 87 per cent at Severalls. One way of estimating a staff–patient ratio is to exclude patients leaving the ward for some form of employment or occupational therapy and also nurses who accompany them. This calculation showed that on the selected wards there were, during a typical day, 10 nurses and 20 patients at Netherne, 8 nurses and 81 patients at Mapperley, and 31 nurses and 488 patients at Severalls. Occupational therapists working on the ward were included in this calculation. At Netherne (and to a lesser extent at Mapperley) far more non-nursing staff helped to care for patients during the day away from the wards. For example, male and female patients worked in the following departments: laundry, tailor's shop, sewing room, bakery, staff cafeteria, works department, printing shop, butcher's, engineers' and fitters', kitchen, offices, garage, fire station, farm, poultry farm, market garden, ornamental garden, sports field, library, salvage department, special paint spray shop for patients, woodwork departments (one specially for patients), two large industrial workshops, two smaller occupational therapy departments, and domestic work in various parts of the hospital (other than the patient's own ward).

When all patients were on the wards, there was very little difference in the average nursing staff–patient ratio at the three hospitals (about 1 nurse to 20 patients during the day shift). The significant difference at Netherne was not better staffing of the wards but a far greater use of nurses, occupational therapists and utility staff to work with patients off the ward. Mapperley showed a similar extension but to a lesser extent; but there was very little for patients at Severalls to do.

Time budget

Table 5.4 (p. 207) gives details of the average time spent, by patients in the three samples, on certain daily tasks. Netherne and Mapperley hospitals are fairly similar. Severalls Hospital differs from them very markedly; in particular, patients spent a great deal of time in the ward on the day covered by the survey (only 30 per cent left the ward at all) and the time spent either doing 'nothing' (5 hours 39 minutes) or at 'toilet' or 'meals' (3 hours 10 minutes) when in the ward is very long compared with the other two hospitals. An average of 68 per cent of the patients' total time out of bed was accounted for under these two headings. (The patient was only regarded as doing 'nothing' when there was no evidence that she was occupied in any way which could possibly be called constructive or leisure activity.) A high score (e.g. nine hours) would be recorded for a patient who remained inert the whole day on the same chair she occupied at breakfast; a lower score (e.g. four hours) by one who did some ward work during the day but after tea sat in a chair until bedtime, neither talking, knitting, reading nor watching television, etc. In case of any doubt, judgement was given against a recording of 'nothing'.

Netherne and Mapperley hospitals differed in two important ways. First, at Mapperley considerably less time was spent in leisure activities (particularly watching television, though this was available on all wards). The explanation appears to be a much earlier bedtime— 7.38 p.m. compared with 8.30 p.m. at Netherne and 8.13 p.m. at Severalls. Secondly, somewhat fewer patients worked for at least three hours per day. 'Work' was defined as occupation in the grounds, or in hospital departments, special industrial work or outside employment, and excluded ordinary occupational therapy. Simply being present in a workshop or department did not, of course, count as work—the patient had to be actively employed.

Figure 5.5 (p. 208) shows the proportion of patients at each hospital who 'did nothing' for five hours or more each day, separately for each clinical category. The main differences between hospitals remain unaffected when clinical group is controlled.

Personal possessions

The main differences appeared between Severalls Hospital and the other two. For example, 33 patients in Severalls had *no* personal possessions at all (44 if items of clothing are not considered), whereas none at Mapperley and only one at Netherne were without any effects at all.

Some detailed results are presented in Figure 5.6 (p. 209). While patients at Netherne and Mapperley hospitals possessed comparable amounts of clothing, Mapperley occupied a more intermediate position when other articles were considered. In figures for possession of a comb, or brush, for instance, Mapperley (69 per cent) occupied an intermediate position between Netherne and Severalls (89 and 45 per cent), while the numbers owning scissors or a nail file at Netherne (55 per cent) far exceeded those at either Mapperley or Severalls (18 and 8 per cent).

Figure 5.7 (p. 210) shows the proportion of patients at each hospital who had no possessions at all, separately for each clinical category.

Nurses' opinions about patients

Ward sisters at Netherne Hospital were more optimistic in their opinions about the patients than those at either Mapperley or Severalls (see Figure 5.8, p. 211). Nurses at Mapperley Hospital tended to be intermediate or to approach those at Severalls Hospital very closely. For example, 76 per cent of patients were thought capable of doing useful work (laundry, domestic work, etc.) for the hospital, compared with 52 per cent at Mapperley and only 26 per cent at Severalls. There was a high degree of agreement between nurses at all three hospitals on only two questions. Few patients were considered to need certification, and few were thought to be fit enough to work outside the hospital while living in.

Figure 5.9 (p. 212) shows the proportion of patients at each hospital who were judged by the ward sister to be capable of useful work. Again, controlling for clinical condition diminishes the differences between hospitals very little.

Differences in the social environments provided

Thus the three hospitals provided quite different social environments for the patients in this study. It is therefore possible to test the hypothesis that the clinical condition of the patients in the three groups should also be different.

MENTAL STATE, WARD BEHAVIOUR AND ATTITUDE TO DISCHARGE

Classification of mental state

Table 5.10 (p. 213) shows that there were significant differences in the distribution of the clinical subgroups at the three hospitals. There were fewer moderately ill patients in the sample from Severalls Hospital (23 per cent compared with 39 per cent in Mapperley Hospital and 40 per cent in Netherne Hospital). On the other hand, there were 56 per cent at Severalls who showed severe flatness of affect or poverty of speech—subgroups 4 and 5—compared with 39 per cent at Mapperley and 26 per cent at Netherne.

There was a significant association between clinical classification and length of stay in hospital ($\chi^2 = 21\cdot71$, df $= 8$, p $< 0\cdot01$). In particular, relatively few patients in subgroups 1 and 2 had been in hospital twenty-one years or more, and relatively few patients in subgroup 5 had been in hospital for less than ten years. Since there were fewer patients at Netherne who had been in hospital twenty-one years or more, or who were aged 51–60, than at the other two hospitals, the age and length of stay distributions at Mapperley and Severalls were standardised to those of Netherne. This reduced the numbers of patients at Mapperley in subgroups 4 and 5 to 32 per cent—very little different to the proportion at Netherne. At Severalls, however, the deficiency of patients in subgroup 1 (26 per cent when corrected) and the excess in subgroups 4 and 5 (51 per cent when corrected) still remained.

Table 5.11 (p. 213) shows that there is no significant association between clinical classification and occupation of patients' fathers. This held true for each of the hospitals taken separately, and also when the non-manual occupations were broken down further into professional, managerial, administrative, supervisory and clerical.

Behaviour in ward

The mean S.W. scores for the samples of patients from Netherne, Mapperley and Severalls were 3·0, 4·6 and 5·5 respectively (F $= 10\cdot0$, p $< 0\cdot001$). Thus patients at Netherne showed least abnormality in this respect. The mean S.E. scores were 1·2, 2·3 and 1·3 respectively (F $= 9\cdot8$, p $< 0\cdot001$): that is, patients at Mapperley showed most disturbance on this scale.

A special check was necessary because 34 per cent of patients in Mapperley and 21 per cent of patients in Severalls came from one large long-stay ward. If the two ward sisters concerned had been unduly severe in their ratings of ward behaviour they could have biassed the comparison with Netherne. Their ratings were therefore compared with ratings made by other ward sisters in the same hospital, and with the mental state ratings made independently by the investigator. There was no indication that a special bias was operating in either case.

Table 5.12 shows mean S.W. and S.E. scores in three length-of-stay groups. Analysis of variance of S.W. scores disclosed very highly significant differences between hospitals and between length-of-stay groups. Subsequent t-tests showed that there was a significant increase in score with length of stay. Patients in Severalls Hospital showed significantly higher mean scores than patients in Netherne Hospital, however long they had been in hospital. However, there was a gradation in mean score at Mapperley Hospital. Patients who had been resident 2–10 years were not significantly different from equivalent patients in Netherne Hospital. Patients who had been resident more than 21 years were not significantly different from equivalent patients in Severalls Hospital. The remaining patients, who had been in hospital 11–20 years, had a mean score which was intermediate between those of equivalent patients in Netherne and Severalls Hospitals.

There was no significant variation in S.E. score with length of stay in hospital.

Mean S.W. and S.E. scores for patients whose fathers were in various occupational groups are shown in Table 5.13 (p. 214). Combining equivalent groups from the three hospitals, there was significant variation in both scores. Subsequent t-tests showed that this was mainly due to the fact that patients whose fathers were skilled manual workers tended to have lower scores than other groups (this was also true of the three hospitals taken separately). There was no tendency for the prestige (according to the Hall Jones scale) of the father's occupation to be associated with the degree of disturbance of the patient's behaviour.

Attitude to discharge

Fifty-four per cent of patients in Netherne Hospital, 66 per cent in Mapperley Hospital and 70 per cent in Severalls Hospital were either indifferent about being discharged or actually wanted to stay ($\chi^2 = 5.81$, p = just over 0.05). There was an association between clinical classification and attitude to discharge. If patients who were indifferent were omitted, 62 per cent of moderately ill patients and patients with coherently expressed delusions (subgroups 1 and 2) had some desire to leave, compared with 49 per cent of the remaining groups. Indifference was, of course, strongly related to poverty of speech and muteness. The relationship between attitude to discharge and length of stay is shown in Table 5.14 (p. 215), which also shows the detailed results for the three hospitals. There was a decrease in the proportion of those wishing to leave, the longer patients had been resident, in each of the three hospitals. When either clinical condition or length of stay was controlled, there was no difference between hospitals.

Drug treatment

One other item of information which was systematically collected for all patients in the samples will be considered here. The ward sisters were asked to say what drug treatment the patients had been receiving during the previous week. The detailed results are presented in Table 5.15 (p. 216).

More patients at Mapperley Hospital were receiving major tranquillisers or sedatives, by day, than at the other two hospitals. In order to provide a direct comparison, doses of the major tranquillisers were translated into arbitrary units, roughly equivalent to 100 mg. of Chlorpromazine. A total of 149 units daily was prescribed for the 100 patients at Netherne, 192 units for the 73 patients at Mapperley (i.e. 262 for 100 patients), and 145 units for the 100 patients at Severalls. Sodium amytal was also prescribed in larger quantities, by day, at Mapperley than at the other two hospitals.

COMPARISON OF MATCHED PATIENTS

Twenty patients at each hospital were selected (without knowledge of their scores on these social measures) because they were equivalent in clinical grouping, S.W. score, S.E. score, age, length of stay in hospital and attitude towards discharge (that is, they were matched triplets). This was relatively simple since several of the variables were correlated. The clinical condition of these patients was considerably above the average for the complete samples. Differences between hospitals, in terms of social measurements, were reduced when only these twenty patients were considered, but for the great majority of items tested large differences still remained between Severalls Hospital and the other two. There was, for example, little difference between the numbers leaving the ward for any reason in Netherne and Mapperley hospitals (17 and 16 respectively), but in Severalls Hospital only 9 had done so. Differences between Netherne and Mapperley tended to be much reduced, but on some items they were still significant. These included certain attitudes of the nursing staff, for example, towards possession of matches, bathing alone, and going out with a male patient, in all of which staff at Mapperley Hospital were more doubtful.

Discussion

The results given in this chapter show a consistent pattern in the three hospitals studied. Netherne and Severalls hospitals provide markedly different social environments according to all the criteria used—ward restrictiveness, time budget, personal possessions and nurses' attitudes, while Mapperley Hospital in some respects is similar to Netherne and in others to Severalls. It was therefore possible to test the hypothesis that there should be parallel clinical differences between the three groups of patients.

In fact, the same pattern is evident in the measurements of mental state and socially withdrawn behaviour. Patients in the sample of female long-stay schizophrenics from Netherne Hospital tend to show least disturbance in verbal behaviour at interview, and least disturbance of social behaviour in the ward (assessed by S.W. score), while patients in the sample from Severalls Hospital tend to show most disturbance on these two variables. Mapperley Hospital patients are intermediate in both respects, though when age and length of stay are allowed for, they approximate more closely to patients in Netherne Hospital so far as verbal behaviour at interview is concerned. The difference in ward behaviour between Netherne and Mapperley patients is confined to those who have been resident over ten years: in this very long-stay group, ward behaviour (S.W. score) is closer to that in Severalls. S.E. scores are significantly higher at Mapperley than at the other two hospitals, particularly in the longer-stay groups. No interpretation of this finding can be offered at this stage of the analysis.

A description of three wards, which provides flesh for the bare bones of the statistical analysis, will be found in Chapter 8. However, this is not relevant at this stage since the main problem of interpretation cannot be answered by descriptive data. The problem can be stated as follows: Are the different social conditions under which the patients live responsible for the differences in their clinical condition in the three hospitals, or are there different processes of selection which ensure that more clinically disturbed patients accumulate in one hospital than in another? If the latter process is operating, the high proportion of severely-ill patients might determine the social and administrative policies of the hospital rather than the other way round. In fact, the extent to which treatment procedures had to be adapted to clinically disturbed patients might lead to generalisation of these procedures to cover even moderately-ill patients. This would account for the fact that differences between the hospitals in respect of personal possessions, ward routines and nurses' opinions persist even within clinical categories, and when age and length of stay have been allowed for.

It might be objected that a patient who was offered the choice of admission to a chronic ward in one of these hospitals in 1960 would have considered this a somewhat academic argument. There is little doubt on the evidence that, though she might have hesitated between Netherne and Mapperley hospitals, she would have rejected Severalls Hospital at once. However, the point at issue is not which hospital provides most comfort for its chronic schizophrenic patients, or which a discriminating patient would most like to live in. The question is: Do the differences in social atmosphere indicate that one hospital will have a beneficial, while another has a harmful, effect on the mental health of its inmates (irrespective of whether they like it there or not)? The answer to this question should not be taken for granted because it seems obvious on humanitarian grounds.

The data collected in the present 'cross-sectional' survey are not very well suited to answering questions of this kind. However, a number of checks may be made, and two kinds of 'longitudinal' data can be gathered which may help to provide an answer. The two alternatives may be taken separately: Does the environment influence the patients, or do the patients create their own environment? In the latter case, it should be possible to demonstrate some kind of selective process at work, above all in Severalls Hospital, to account for the high proportion of clinically disturbed patients there. Two possibilities suggest themselves. The social class structure of the three communities is very different and possibly a different type of patient is being admitted to Severalls Hospital. This argument cannot be carried very far, since Mapperley Hospital admits from an area which is similar in social class; and, in any case, clinical classification and ward behaviour are not related to the occupation of the patients' fathers. The case-notes of all schizophrenic patients entering the three hospitals have been studied and rated, and no evidence was found that Severalls admitted more severely ill patients. Another possibility is that there is a relatively high early discharge rate in Severalls, so that the severely-ill patients, with a bad prognosis, who remain and accumulate in the hospital, would form a high proportion of all patients who had been resident for more than two years. Alternatively, there might be a specially high number of discharges of moderately-ill chronic patients from Severalls, with the same result. The latter suggestion has been checked and it is found that Netherne had had by far the highest annual discharge rate of chronic schizo-phrenic patients during the previous ten years. Mapperley retained its schizophrenic patients admitted in 1956 for the shortest time, while Netherne and Severalls were similar in this respect (Brown *et al.*, 1966).

If anything, therefore, these results seem to point in the opposite direction. But even if there had been a specially high early discharge rate at Severalls, which distinguished it from the other hospitals, it is not clear that this would necessarily mean an accumulation of a large proportion of severely-ill patients. Mapperley had the lowest pro-portion of patients retained for two years, of the three hospitals, but 39 per cent of the long-stay schizophrenics were moderately ill. Thus, not only severely-ill patients are retained (and, probably, not only moderately-ill patients are discharged).

There was a further method of checking the selection hypothesis. If the survey could be repeated in the three hospitals, after the lapse of a suitable period of time, using the same individuals, selective factors would be held constant. Any changes that had taken place in clinical condition would therefore be attributable either to the lapse of time alone or to the introduction of changes in social conditions or in physical treatment. Most of the patients were already receiving adequate doses of the new tranquillising drugs and no major development in this direction has taken place. A definite test of the general hypothesis is therefore possible, and the results will be presented in Chapters 6 and 7.

Summary

1. Social differences between hospitals in 1960 were evident both in matters of central importance in everyday life and in small details. For example, there was a 50 per cent difference between Netherne and Severalls hospitals in the proportion of the sample leaving the ward during the day, and a 60 per cent difference in the proportion of patients possessing a toothbrush. Severalls patients, on average, spent 5 hours 39 minutes of their waking time doing absolutely nothing, compared with 2 hours 48 minutes at Netherne. Mapperley Hospital, on the whole, approximated to Netherne Hospital, but also showed certain similarities to Severalls Hospital. In matters of obvious importance, such as the amount of time spent off the ward, the opportunities for constructive work, the provision of respectable personal clothing, the amount of locker space, etc., Mapperley Hospital was more or less equivalent to Netherne Hospital. But in more intimate, and perhaps less obvious, details, the patients at Mapperley were not so well off as those at Netherne. Fewer patients, for example, possessed scissors or a mirror, and fewer baths were 'screened' from onlookers. Patients went to bed on average nearly one hour before those at Netherne and leisure activities were more restricted. These differences were further reflected in the opinions of the nursing staff. Ward sisters thought, at Mapperley, that *all* patients should be helped to buy clothing and, at Netherne, that 91 per cent of patients should. On the other hand they thought, at Mapperley, that only 27 per cent of patients could be trusted with matches, while Netherne ward sisters said that 79 per cent of patients were trustworthy in this way.

2. There were differences between the hospitals in respect of the age, length of stay, and social class composition of the samples of long-stay schizophrenic patients studied. When these were allowed for, there was little difference in the clinical classification of the samples from Netherne and Mapperley hospitals, but Severalls Hospital contained significantly more severely impaired patients. For example, 24 per cent of the patients in Severalls were mute at interview, but only 6 per cent at Netherne. Ward behaviour was significantly more characterised by social withdrawal at Mapperley and Severalls than at Netherne. Patients at Mapperley, according to

the S.W. scores, behaved like those from Netherne before they had been in hospital ten years, and like those from Severalls in the longer-stay groups. S.E. scores, on the other hand, were highest at Mapperley.

In general, the sample from Netherne showed least disturbance in verbal behaviour at interview, and in ward behaviour, while the sample from Severalls showed most. Patients in Mapperley were in some respects like the former, in some respects like the latter.

3. When twenty patients from each hospital, matched in respect of clinical condition, length of stay and attitude to discharge, were compared, the great majority of social measurements still showed a similar pattern of differences between the hospitals.

4. In all three hospitals, attitudes to discharge became more unfavourable the longer patients had been resident. When clinical condition or length of stay were controlled, there was no difference between hospitals in the overall proportion of patients with un-favourable attitudes.

5. More patients at Mapperley were receiving major tranquillisers, in larger doses, than at the other two hospitals. Patients at Netherne and Severalls were receiving much the same amount of medication so that the clinical differences between their in-patients cannot be ascribed to differences in drug treatment.

6. Alternative explanations for these findings are discussed.

6

CHANGES IN PATIENTS AND
ENVIRONMENT, 1960–1964

The surveys were repeated in 1962 at Mapperley and Severalls and in 1964 at all three hospitals, exactly two years and four years after the initial investigations. All the patients who were still in hospital were re-interviewed and the same social and behavioural measurements made. Usually, the nurses who completed questionnaires or who gave information to the sociologist about any particular patient were not the same, even for two out of three possible occasions of measurement.

The person who enumerated the patient's personal possessions was different on each occasion. The investigators never looked up their notes of previous interviews or observations at the time of making new ones. Although, in certain instances, it was possible to remember roughly what the previous measurements had been (particularly in the third surveys at Mapperley and Severalls), in general, contamination from this source was likely to be low during the second surveys.

Stated simply, the hypotheses under test in this chapter are that, if environmental conditions improved, symptoms such as flatness of affect, poverty of speech and social withdrawal should also have improved, and clinical change should occur most frequently in those patients whose social milieu had changed. Florid symptoms would be less likely to improve in association with decreased poverty of the social environment, and attitudes to discharge should not, on balance, change at all. Any clinical improvement observed would be independent of changes in the type or dose of phenothiazines prescribed.

This chapter is concerned solely with the overall differences found between the two surveys of 1960 and 1964. Changes within each of the three hospitals are compared in Chapter 7, which also presents data collected in 1962 and January 1968.

OUTCOME IN 1964

Of the 273 patients who were interviewed in 1960, 40 had been discharged, transferred to another hospital or had died, by the time of the surveys in 1964. Since outcome is discussed in Chapter 7, on the basis of the follow-up in January 1968, no further consideration will be given to these 40 patients here. The analysis in this chapter concerns the remaining 233 patients, all of whom were in one of the three hospitals in 1964. Two had been discharged and re-admitted but they are not separated from the rest in the analysis.

SOCIAL CHANGES, 1960–1964

The scores on all six measures of poverty of the social environment show that an improvement occurred between 1960 and 1964 (see Table 6.1, p. 217).

The order of improvement is understood more clearly if some of these scores are considered in more detail. Nurses' attitudes, for example, are summarised in Table 6.2 (p. 217). Attitudes are shown in four categories. The first category contains three attitudes which were favourable even in 1960, and were more favourable still in 1964. The fourth category contains two attitudes which remained very unfavourable throughout. The other two categories contain attitudes which were intermediate in 1960 between those in the first and the fourth categories: both groups show considerable improvement in 1964. The second category is composed of relatively 'neutral' attitudes, to money, work in hospital and shopping, while the third category contains attitudes which indicate a considerable degree of responsibility for personal behaviour being allowed to the patient (possessing matches or scissors, bathing alone, going out with men). The first three improve roughly to the same extent considering the room there is for improvement. The fourth improves hardly at all, although there is much room for improvement.

These attitudes on the part of nurses do not, of course, necessarily represent their actual behaviour. Some check on this is given by the data in Table 6.3 (p. 218), which summarise the increase in personal ownership of clothes and toilet materials. In 1964, nearly every patient owned 'obvious' items such as a dress, overcoat or hair-brush, a fact which actually runs ahead of the improvement in the nurses' attitudes (in 1964, nurses thought that 89 per cent of the patients could own their own clothing). Similarly the order of improvement in the ownership of items such as handbags and personal ornaments is equivalent to the improvement in the nurses' attitudes towards the patients' expected performance with money and shopping. Nevertheless, even in 1964, 20 per cent of patients owned neither a purse nor a handbag; equipment which helps to make a woman's performance of her social role more convincing. The possession of possibly dangerous items like matches, scissors or nail files only increased by 9 per cent, and still remained the exception in 1964, whereas the nurses' expressed opinions, both in 1960 and in 1964, were very much more favourable in their assumption that patients could responsibly own such things.

The change in patients' activities between 1960 and 1964 is shown in more detail in Table 6.4 (p. 218). There was a decrease of one hour in the mean time doing nothing (from four-and-a-half to three-and-a-half hours), accounted for mainly by an increase in work and in leisure activities.

Increase in amount of contact with the outside world was less impressive than improvement in the other measures, but not negligible. Twenty patients were much better off in this respect, and 40 patients somewhat better off, compared with 8 patients whose contact decreased markedly and 23 whose contact decreased somewhat. The remaining 142 patients did not experience any great change.

Ward restrictiveness score could only be directly compared for 135 patients, of whom 80 (59 per cent) remained in a ward of roughly the same degree of restrictiveness or liberality as before. Ten patients were actually worse off and the remaining 45 (33 per cent) were in less restrictive environments.

Further details concerning occupation, outside contact and ward restrictiveness are given in Chapter 7.

The interrelationships between these variables, and with length of stay, remained much the same as in 1960 (see Tables 4.1 and 4.2, pp. 199 and 200). That is to say, the conclusions reached in Chapter 4, regarding poverty of the social environment and length of stay, remain true in the 1964 data.

Thus, in summary, the social conditions under which patients were living had improved considerably between 1960 and 1964. Nurses' attitudes were more favourable, personal possessions had increased, ward restrictiveness had lessened, working and leisure activities were commoner at the expense of time spent doing nothing, and there was a little more contact with the outside world. If our hypothesis is correct, poverty of clinical condition should also have improved and, most important of all, it should specifically have been the patients who experienced better social conditions who made most progress.

CLINICAL CHANGES, 1960–1964

Table 6.5 (p. 219) shows that there was, indeed, an improvement in clinical condition, as measured by the overall categorisation, in about one-third of patients. Seventy-three out of 133 patients (31 per cent) were moderately handicapped, according to these criteria, both in 1960 and in 1964 (Group M). Seventy-one (31 per cent) were severely handicapped in 1960 but had improved by at least one category in 1964 (Group I). This includes 4 patients who showed predominantly severe incoherence of speech instead of severe poverty of speech. The remaining 89 patients (Group NC) had not changed (N = 79) or actually became worse (N = 10). (These three groups are used, for convenience, in much of the rest of the analysis in this book.) It is worth remarking that there was no change of category in 150 patients out of 233, to which should probably be added 20 out of the 24 patients who were discharged before the time of the 1964 survey, and all the patients who were transferred or who died, making roughly two-thirds of the original 273 patients, who showed no major change in clinical condition.

This operational technique of measuring improvement in clinical category is based upon the clinical categorisation made at the time of the two interviews in 1960 and 1964. When the actual protocols were subsequently compared, some of the changes were difficult to demonstrate in the written notes, though they might, of course, have been validly based on impressions (for example, of affective contact) which were too subtle to record. In perhaps 21 of the 71 cases of 'improvement' the documented change (apart from the ratings) was rather small: the social withdrawal score in these cases dropped from 3·09 to 2·74; an insignificant decrease. In a further 26 cases the change was clearly evident from the written records and in the remaining 24 there was a very marked and obvious recorded improvement. The social withdrawal score for these 50 patients decreased from 6·04 to 3·62, which is highly significant. The four examples of notes taken at the time of interview, which are given in

Appendix 6.1, illustrate the order of improvement represented in these 50 patients.

Thus 50 out of 233 patients (21 per cent) could confidently be said to have improved clinically, while another 21 may well have done so but there is only the clinician's judgement for evidence. It will be shown in Chapter 7 that patients who improved clinically according to the clinical ratings were more likely to be discharged.

The degree of improvement in the four clinical symptoms (flatness of affect, poverty of speech, incoherence of speech and coherently-expressed delusions) taken separately, is shown in Table 6.6 (p. 219), from which it is clear that the two 'negative' symptoms show most improvement.

Analysing the change in the 64 patients with severe florid symptoms in 1960, 23 (36 per cent) had symptoms of only moderate severity in 1964, 36 (56 per cent) still had severe florid symptoms and the remaining 5 (8 per cent) now had severe negative symptoms. Of the 93 patients with severe negative symptoms in 1960, 26 (28 per cent) had symptoms of only moderate severity in 1964, 12 (13 per cent) developed severe florid symptoms, and 55 (59 per cent) remained unchanged. Thus there seems to be no evidence for a progression from negative through florid symptoms as the patient improved, although the long period of time between ratings would not necessarily show this up.

The relationship between clinical improvement category derived from ratings made by the psychiatrist and the S.W. score (derived from the nurses' ratings) are shown in Tables 6.7 and 6.8 (p. 220). There is a highly significant 'groups by occasions' interaction, showing that the two techniques pick out substantially similar groups of improved patients.

The detailed changes in behaviour are shown in Table 6.9 (p. 221), from which it is clear that most symptoms improved to some extent though the overall change was not very great. The low degree of serious disturbance in behaviour is illustrated by the fact that only 5 per cent of patients were incontinent (and 22 per cent needed supervision) during the sample week and only 4 per cent were violent (and 16 per cent were threatening in behaviour).

The clinical improvement groups are not significantly related to age, marital status or father's occupation in 1960, but there is a significant association with length of stay. Considering groups I and NC only, nearly 70 per cent of patients in hospital for twenty-one years or more show no improvement or even get worse, compared with roughly half the patients with a shorter stay (see Table 6.10, p. 221).

Table 6.9 shows that there is an overall improvement in florid symptomatology. Indeed, patients whose predominant symptom is coherently-expressed delusions are most likely, of all the severely-impaired groups, to show improvement. Fourteen out of twenty-three did so, while only one deteriorated. Patients with incoherence of speech, on the other hand, are least likely to show an improvement.

Since the negative symptoms and syndromes are commoner than the florid ones, the amelioration in the latter does not stand out clearly, but it is definitely there and our hypothesis to the contrary is disproven.

INTERACTION BETWEEN SOCIAL AND CLINICAL CHANGES, 1960–1964

The crucial test of our hypothesis linking decreased poverty of the social environment to decreased poverty of clinical condition, lies in the attempt to discover whether patients who have been exposed to the changed milieu improve, while patients who have not been so exposed do not improve. The two groups I and NC are conveniently compared for this purpose, since patients in both groups showed severe speech disorder in 1960, but those in group I improved clinically while those in group NC did not.

Table 6.11 (p. 222) shows the mean score in 1960, and the mean change in score from 1960 to 1964, on five measures of poverty of the social environment, for the three clinical improvement groups separately. Analyses of variance were carried out on each variable. In each case there was a very highly significant improvement between occasions. On all variables except occupation, there was also a very highly significant difference between groups in 1960: on occupation, the significance was at the 1 per cent level. Most of the difference was accounted for by the better scores of group M in 1960. In one case, however, group I had a higher mean score on personal possessions in 1960 than had group NC ($t = 2.2$, $df = 237$, $p < 0.05$). The significance of any changes in score between 1960 and 1964 is shown in the table. Comparing groups I and NC only, two scores show very highly significant improvement in both: nurses' attitudes and personal possessions. In the case of personal possessions, however, there is a highly significant interaction, and group I improves very significantly more than group NC. The other three scores (outside contact, occupation and time doing nothing) show a significant improvement only for group I. In the case of outside contact, there is no significant interaction overall—however group I does show a highly significant improvement compared with group NC. The groups by occasions interaction is significant for occupation (p < 0·01) and time doing nothing (p < 0·001) and, in both cases, there is a very highly significant improvement in the mean score of group I, and virtually no change in the mean score of group NC.

In summary, groups I and NC are fairly closely matched on the five social variables in 1960 and both score less favourably than group M. The improvement shown by group NC patients is less than that shown by group I patients, on all measures. However, both groups improve very considerably on personal possessions and nurses' attitudes, while improvement on occupation and time doing nothing is virtually confined to group I. Improvement on outside contact, though greater in group I than in group NC, is less impressive than the improvement on the other scores.

In order to compare the change in amount of time doing nothing with, on the one hand, change in clinical category and, on the other, change in social withdrawal score, three groups were set up:

Group X: patients with a score of under 2 hours in 1960 *and* in 1964 (i.e. they spent less than two hours doing nothing according to both ratings);

Group Y: patients who scored 2·0+ hours in 1960, whose scores decreased by 2·0 hours or more in 1964;

Group Z: patients who scored 2·0+ hours in 1960, whose score did *not* decrease by 2·0 hours or more in 1964, or whose score increased.

Tables 6.12 and 6.13 (pp. 222 and 223) show the relationship between improvement in time doing nothing and the two measures of clinical condition. In each case there is a significant relationship between clinical improvement and decrease in time doing nothing, in those groups where there was room for improvement. The relationship with clinical category is particularly striking.

There is no association between groups X, Y and Z and length of stay, age, marital status or father's occupation.

Finally, the time budget of daily activities is set out in more detail in Table 6.14 (p. 223), for the three clinical improvement groups. The only positive improvement that characterises patients in group I is an increase in time devoted to work and occupational therapy (1·8 hours compared with 0·2 hours in group NC): the outstanding change is a decrease in time doing nothing (2·7 hours compared with 0·5 hours). An increase in time spent watching television or listening to the radio, or in other leisure activities, does not seem to be specially related to clinical improvement.

CHANGE IN ATTITUDES TO DISCHARGE, 1960–1964

On the basis of the findings detailed in Chapter 4, it is hypothesised that attitudes to discharge are unlikely to improve very markedly. Table 6.15 (p. 224) gives the figures, which broadly confirm the hypothesis. Of the 165 patients who were rated on both occasions, 27 improved in attitude (from a rating of 4 or 5 to one of 1, 2 or 3), 24 adopted a less favourable attitude (being rated 4 or 5 instead of 1, 2 or 3), and 114 did not change their views. Taking a more strict criterion, only 10 patients changed from being indifferent or wanting to stay (or being unrateable) to definitely wanting to leave (a rating of 1 or 2); and only 5 changed in the opposite direction—making a total of 15 definite changes in all.

From Figure 4.4 (p. 202) it is possible to calculate that, each year before 1960, roughly 2·2 per cent of long-stay patients changed their attitudes, from wishing to leave (ratings of 1, 2 or 3) to being indifferent or wishing to stay. Thus 9 per cent would be expected to change in this way between 1960 and 1964 and, in fact, nearly 15 per cent did so. However, 16 per cent changed in the opposite direction so that there was no net difference. The relationship between length of stay and attitude to discharge remained marked in 1964, but it is interesting to note that the proportion of patients in the longest-stay group, who wished to leave, increased in 1964 (Table 6.16, p. 224).

A further analysis of patients who changed their attitudes yielded few associations of interest, except that there was a non-significant tendency for patients who were less ill in 1960 to change towards wanting to stay, and *vice versa*.

PHENOTHIAZINES

The dose (and change in dose) of phenothiazines was examined within the three clinical improvement groups (M, I and NC), the three groups formed on the basis of social withdrawal scores (D, E and F), and the three groups formed on the basis of 'time doing nothing' in 1960 and 1964 (X, Y and Z). No associations of significance were observed, but the overall dose of phenothiazine increased a little in all groups during the four years.

Discussion

The data presented in this chapter provide more solid evidence that certain social and clinical events are causally interrelated. Poverty of the social environment *did* lessen between the 1960 and 1964 surveys and poverty of clinical condition decreased concomitantly. Since not all patients improved clinically, it was possible to compare those who showed severe symptoms at the initial survey, and who subsequently appeared less socially withdrawn or had less speech disorder, with those who did not improve in these ways. Clinical improvement occurred significantly more often in patients whose social environment had improved. Although all the indices of social milieu showed improvement, a reduction in the amount of time doing nothing appeared to be far and away the most important index associated with clinical progress.

Discussion of the alternative hypotheses which might explain these results will be withheld until other relevant data have been presented.

As was predicted from the data presented in Chapter 4, there was little overall change in the proportions of patients wishing to leave hospital in 1960 and 1964. However, the deterioration in attitude and length of stay was balanced by the adoption of more favourable attitudes by certain patients who had previously been indifferent or who wished to remain in hospital. Although the conclusion is not certain, it is possible that there is more likelihood of change in attitudes which were formerly resistant to change, when social improvements are introduced. In the absence of a specific attempt to change attitudes, this might work both ways—more patients being likely to adopt unfavourable attitudes as well as more changing to a positive wish for discharge.

Further information bearing on these matters, and on more practical questions of how the social environments of hospitals change, is discussed in Chapter 7, which deals with differences between the three hospitals in 1964 compared with 1960, and introduces material collected in 1962 and January 1968.

Summary

1. Forty patients had been discharged, transferred to another hospital or had died between 1960 and 1964. The analysis in this chapter is based on the results obtained for the remaining 233 patients.

2. There was a significant improvement on all six measures of the social environment when results for 1960 and 1964 were compared. Nurses' attitudes were more favourable, personal possessions had increased, ward restrictiveness had lessened, working and leisure activities were commoner at the expense of time doing nothing, and there was a little more contact with the outside world.

3. About one-third of the patients improved somewhat in clinical condition—in 21 per cent the improvement was quite definite. The 'negative' symptoms—flatness of affect, poverty of speech and social withdrawal—all showed change. Coherently-expressed delusions also improved, while incoherence of speech and socially embarrassing behaviour were less affected.

4. Seventy-one patients, who were severely impaired in 1960 but had improved by 1964, were compared with 89 patients who were severely impaired on both occasions. Two social measures showed a marked change for the better in both groups—favourable nurses' attitudes and personal possessions. They were therefore unlikely to have caused the clinical improvement, which occurred in only one group. Contact with the outside increased to some extent in clinically improved patients and not at all in unimproved patients. The main difference between those who were clinically better in 1964 compared with those who showed no change was in occupation score and, particularly, a decrease in time doing nothing (5·7 to 3·0 hours compared with 5·4 to 4·9 hours).

5. Attitudes to discharge changed very little during the four years, in spite of the social and clinical improvements.

6. There was no association between change in dose or type of medication and clinical improvement.

APPENDIX 6.1

Four case-summaries of patients who improved according to repeated clinical ratings, where the improvement was also demonstrable in the clinical notes made at the time of interview. In each case, the four clinical ratings are given in the same order: flatness of affect, poverty of speech, incoherence of speech, coherently-expressed delusions.

NETHERNE PATIENT NO. 98

1960 interview

How long have you been here? *Not very long.*
How do you like it? *All right.*
Do you want to leave hospital? *No, it's all right.*
Would you be content to stay? *Yes.*
Permanently? *I don't know.*

    (Rating of attitude to discharge, 5; wants to stay.)

What are your chances of settling down outside? (No reply.)
Have you any relatives come to visit? *All of them.*
How do you mean? (No reply.)
Who comes to see you? (No reply.)

(The remainder of the interview was much like this. The patient was neat and clean with a 'pudding basin' haircut and no make-up. Her answers were monosyllabic and she could give no details, even of the money she received each week. Her affect was severely flattened and could best be described as an indifferent contentment. She sat almost motionless, with her mouth open, and gave an inappropriate smile each time she spoke. Clinical ratings, 4411, Group 4.)

1964 interview

Have you seen me before? *I was just wondering.*
How long have you been in hospital? *A good many years.*
How do you like it? *You get used to it. You have to. I like it all right.*
Do you want to leave? *I wouldn't mind going to see my mother. Get transferred up there. It's only her. I haven't seen my husband for a long time.*
You mean move to a hospital near there? *Yes. I'd love to see my mother.*
What are your chances of getting a job outside? *I don't know. I'm getting on a bit. I might be able to do some housework.*
Would you be content to stay in hospital? *Yes. I want to know how she is.*
To stay permanently? *If I have to.*

    (Rating of attitude to discharge, 5; wants to stay.)

(Patient was able to give a fair account of how she spent her time in hospital—going for a walk each evening, attending the film show, occasional visits to Croydon, watching television occasionally. She was well oriented and could remember some items of recent news. Her affect was moderately flat, her face rather set and her voice rather unvarying, but none of these symptoms was severe. Clinical ratings, 3111, Group 1 *b*.)

MAPPERLEY PATIENT NO. 5

1960 interview

(Patient was muttering quietly to herself as she came into the room and continued to do so throughout the interview, interpolating a few brief answers only.)

How long have you been here? *Two years, I think.*
How do you like it? *I like it all right.*
Do you want to leave? *No, not just yet.*
Would you be content to stay? *Yes.*
Permanently? *Mm.* (Mutters to herself and picks finger nails. Holds a cigarette stub.)
Have you any plans for what you might do outside? *No, I haven't said anything.* (Trails off into audible muttering.)
Do any relatives come to see you? *One or two aunts.*
What work could you do? *No, I don't do any work.*

(Rating of attitude to discharge, 5; wants to stay.)

(The rest of the interview was like this: very brief, vague answers trailing off into muttering. Questions sometimes had to be repeated because patient did not attend to what was said. There was almost no rapport between interviewer and patient, and affect was rated as severely blunted. Personal appearance was nevertheless smart and harmonious though the patient had too much make-up on—it was slightly smeared on her nose—and her powder was not uniformly applied. Her hair was attractively styled. Clinical ratings, 5411, Group 4.)

1962 interview

(Comes into room muttering to herself.)
Do you remember seeing me before? *No, I can't remember.*
How long have you been in hospital? *Three years.*
How do you like it? *I like it all right.*
Do you want to leave? *No, not particularly.*
Would you be content to stay? *Yes.*
Does anyone come to see you? *Sister.*
Anyone else? *Brother.*
How often do they come? *Every few weeks.*

(Rating of attitude to discharge, 5; wants to stay.)

(A large woman wearing too much make-up, rather badly applied. Hair pleasantly styled. Mutters to herself as she comes into the room but then stops and confines herself to a few brief off-putting answers. Occasionally affects not to hear questions or replies only with 'Mm'. Sniffing constantly.

8

Clinical ratings, 4411, Group 4. In retrospect, this patient's speech had already begun to improve somewhat but the rating of 4 still applied. There was a definite improvement in rapport.)

1964 interview

Have you seen me before? *No, I don't remember.*
How long have you been here? *About four years.*
How do you like it? *I don't know. It's all right.*
Do you want to leave? *No, I hadn't thought of leaving.*
Would you be content to stay? *Yes, it's all right here.*
    (Rating of attitude to discharge, 5; wants to stay.)
Does anybody visit you? *Yes, my sister-in-law and brother. They live out Derby way.*
Could you stay with them? *I don't know. I haven't asked them.*
What do you do with your time? *I usually get up in the mornings and do one or two bits; do the laundry, empty the breakfast trolley, clean the room and the toilets and then I don't do anything in the afternoon. I put the cloth on for tea.*
Could you do any work outside? *I don't know what to say. I'm quite happy here.*

(The patient was somewhat overweight. She was smart in appearance and her lipstick was properly applied. She showed definite vagueness in conversation but answered readily and spontaneously. She did not mutter to herself at all and rapport, though superficial, was fair. Clinical ratings, 3311, Group 1 *b*.)

SEVERALLS PATIENT NO. 16

1960 interview

(The patient said she had been in hospital ten years but after that gave no further verbal response. She held her arms in an uncomfortable posture in front of her and she scarcely moved. Her appearance was tidy but she had a fixed gloomy expression, with downward curving lines at each corner of her mouth. Rating of attitude to discharge, 4; indifferent. Clinical ratings, 5511, Group 5.)

1962 interview

Do you remember seeing me before? *No.*
How long have you been here? (No reply.)
A long time? *Yes, rather a long time.*
How do you like it? *I think it's very nice.*
Do you want to leave? (No reply.)
Would you be content to stay? (No reply.)
    (Rating of attitude to discharge, 4; indifferent.)
Have you any relatives come to see you? *Yes, mother used to come.*
Could you do any work outside hospital? *Yes.*

What? *Don't know.*
Do you ever go into town? *Yes, I been out to town once or twice. It was very nice there.*

(The patient whispered to herself at times. There were long pauses before she answered questions and sometimes there was no answer even when questions were repeated, though there were lip movements as if the patient was preparing to answer. Her appearance was not at all smart, with no make-up, institutional dress and haircut. There was little rapport at interview and patient did not respond to a smile. Clinical ratings, 4411, Group 4.)

1964 interview

Do you remember seeing me before? *No.*
How long have you been here? *Don't know.*
How do you like it here? *Nicely, thank you.*
Do you want to leave? *I want to go home. I been on holiday five days.*
Have you any plans? *Stay at home and help me sisters. Three are married and me single.*
How strongly do you feel about leaving? *I don't particularly want to leave unless I go home.*
Would you be content to stay? *Yes, I think so, thank you very much.*
Permanently? *I don't know.*

(Rating of attitude to discharge, 3; ambivalent.)

(Definite flattening of affect but not severe. Able to carry on a conversation and make some spontaneous remarks. Overweight but fair appearance. Clinical ratings, 3311, Group 1*b*.)

SEVERALLS PATIENT NO. 30

1960 interview

How long have you been here? *Oh, years.*
How do you like it? *I can't say I like it at all. I had a day at Frimpinton (?) and the refectory. I never saw such jewels in all my life. Extensive they were. And the cure. The thought operation I had.*
Do you want to leave? *I do please.*
How strongly do you feel about it? *Desperate.*
Would you be content to stay? *No.*
Have you any plans? *No, only to go home.*
Have you any relatives? *A husband and three children. I don't know if he has a person.*
Would he welcome you? *No, he wouldn't.*
Have you somewhere to live? *I wouldn't get in his way. Things are arranged. He always did do the arranging.*
In what way? *He would leave some money.*
What about work? *Not to work. It isn't so strong as that. The words are against creeds and differences. I wouldn't mind.*

(Rating of attitude to discharge, 2; wants to leave but unrealistic.)

(Ordinary but not smart appearance, no make-up. Affect mostly inappropriate or flat. Markedly incoherent speech but also rather vague. Some 'institutional' delusions—for example, that husband and children come weekly to the hospital in a car and bring her money. Clinical ratings, 4343, Group 3.)

1962 interview

Have you seen me before? *A sort of gentleman very similar.*

How long have you been in hospital? *I only came for 4½ months. I got better in 4 months and I haven't really noticed the time. (Rubbing hands together throughout.)*

How do you like it? *I don't like it at all but we do have a walk in the morning. But in the winter it's far too cold.*

Do you want to leave? *Yes.*

How strongly do you feel about it? *I always have felt very strongly about it.*

Would you be content to stay? *No.*

Have you any plans? *To be a housewife and things I'd do.*

Have you any relatives? *Well, yes, I have a certain amount of relatives.*

Would they welcome you? *Go into the house and welcome you home. Don't usually make this amount of fuss in a family. It's still rather extra.*

Have you somewhere to live? *Yes, my home.*

What work would you do? *A clerk.*

Can you get this work? *I think so. Don't see why not.*

How would you set about it? *Answer adverts. in the 'Daily Telegraph' or go to Biddy Montague's—a staff service place.*

How much could you earn? *£2.*

Is that enough? *It doesn't usually absolutely support you. I hadn't thought of that.*

(Rating of attitude to discharge, 2; wants to leave but unrealistic.)

(A thin woman, with lips tightly compressed. Smart appearance with attractively styled hair and no make-up. Moderately flat affect. Delusions only present on direct enquiry, not mentioned spontaneously. Definite examples of incoherence of speech and neologisms but these are not present in spontaneous speech, only when special enquiry is made, e.g.:

Can you think quite clearly? *Yes.*

Any interference with your thoughts? *Oh not any interference or* SLUTTERING.

Anything like hypnotism or telepathy or rays? *I'm too* MURLED. *More of a fixture. It isn't paralysis, mind paralysis. Being here so long that I've got like it. I did work it out once but for the life of me I've forgotten it. It was unbearable but it's going away now.*

How does it affect you? *I think something that I don't think sometimes. Or say something to myself that I hadn't thought at all. It's the condition of being. When I assert myself, it goes.*

No other delusions or incoherence elicited. Clinical ratings, 3133, Group 1*b*.)

1964 interview

Do you remember seeing me before? *A faint resemblance.*
How long have you been here? *A long time.*
How do you like it? *I like this ward better but I don't like hospital.*
Do you want to leave? *I do.*
How strongly do you feel about it? *Very strongly indeed.*
Would you be content to stay? *Oh no.*
Do you think you could get work? *I suppose so.*
What kind? *I'd like a job as a clerk.*
How would you set about getting one? *I don't know.*
Could you support yourself? *Well perhaps I couldn't.*
What about somewhere to stay? *I don't know, I haven't got a home.*

(Rating of attitude to discharge, 2; wants to leave but no plans.)

(Patient's appearance was average; no make-up. Fair rapport and affect.
Speech normal and no evidence of incoherence or delusions even on direct
questioning. Clinical ratings, 3111, Group 1*b*.)

7

CHANGES IN THE THREE HOSPITALS COMPARED, 1960–1968

It was assumed that social and clinical changes after 1960 would be most marked at Severalls, where the room for improvement was greatest, and least marked at Netherne. An analysis of the changes at the hospitals will not only show whether this hypothesis is correct, and whether all differences have been removed by 1964, but it will also afford an opportunity to discover whether the interactions between social and clinical change hold true for each hospital taken separately, which would add greatly to their substance. The first part of this chapter is concerned with these matters. The second part includes material collected in 1962 and in 1968, on the basis of which the time relationships of changes in social conditions and clinical state will be discussed.

Changes within each hospital, 1960–1964

SOCIAL CHANGES IN THE THREE HOSPITALS, 1960–1964

The changes shown by the summary scores on five environmental variables are shown in Table 7.1 (p. 225). At Netherne, personal possessions had increased and outside contact was greater. Although the decrease in hours doing nothing did not reach significance, there is a significant improvement in occupation score. At Mapperley, the nurses' attitudes were more favourable but there was a decrease in personal possessions. At Severalls, there was a very highly significant improvement on all five scores. The amount of time spent doing nothing was still higher than at the other two hospitals in 1964, and the amount of contact with the outside was still less. However, the social environment provided by Severalls in 1964 was little different from that at Mapperley.

Figure 7.2 (p. 225) presents these results in graphic form. The marked improvement at Severalls, according to all five social variables, is clearly shown. It is also clear that Netherne retains its overall lead in 1964 even though Severalls has narrowed the gap in certain respects.

Changes in nurses' attitudes are presented in more detail in Table 7.3 (p. 227). The attitudes are grouped, as in Chapter 6, into four categories. Severalls nurses were much more inclined to think that patients should have their own clothes in 1964, compared with 1960, and the first group of three attitudes showed very little difference between the three hospitals at the time of the 1964 survey. The second group of four attitudes concerning money, work and shopping outside, showed improvement in all hospitals, roughly inversely proportional to the original percentage of favourable attitudes in 1960, so that there were smaller differences between hospitals in 1964, though the same differential was still retained to some extent. A similar process occurred in the third group of attitudes, concerned with potentially dangerous or embarrassing activities. In 1960, nurses at Mapperley and Severalls had been much less favourable in their attitudes than nurses at Netherne, but the difference was much decreased in 1964. The fourth group of attitudes, concerned with working outside hospital or discharge, showed very little change in any hospital—there was no optimism on these points.

A similar detailed analysis of the changes in ownership of various personal articles is shown in Table 7.4 (p. 227). By 1964, practically all patients, in all three hospitals, owned 'obvious' things like a dress or overcoat. There was an all round increase in the ownership of less obvious articles, such as handbags and toothbrushes so that, although the rank order of the hospitals remained the same as in 1960, the differences were much smaller. However, fewer Mapperley patients owned make-up materials or personal ornaments than in 1960, while many more Severalls patients did so. It was striking that two-thirds of the Netherne patients owned potentially dangerous articles such as mirrors and scissors in 1964, while only a quarter did so at Severalls and an even smaller proportion at Mapperley.

A detailed time budget is shown in Table 7.5 (p. 228). There is very little change at Netherne and Mapperley, but a most striking increase in the amount of time engaged in work or occupational therapy at Severalls (an average of 1 hour 48 minutes more per individual) and in leisure activities of various kinds (an increase of 42 minutes, on average, per patient). These changes account for the large decrease in the amount of time spent doing nothing by Severalls patients (a decrease of 2 hours 36 minutes).

Table 7.6 (p. 228) shows the number of patients said by the nurses to be working outside hospital, working in sheltered industrial workshops within the hospital, and either unemployed or doing no more than a little ward work, in 1960 and 1964. The large decrease in Severalls patients who had virtually no occupation at all is very striking. This is largely due to the introduction of industrial work.

Some of the changes in the pattern of contact with the outside world can be seen in Table 7.7 (p. 229). In particular, there was a dramatic increase in the proportion of patients leaving the ward at Severalls, although the number going home did not increase as it did at Netherne.

The changes in ward restrictiveness score are presented in Table 7.8 (p. 229). Only those patients whose wards were rated both in 1960 and in 1964 are included (N = 135). The number of Netherne patients in high-restrictiveness wards has substantially decreased and only 3 out of 51 remain in high-restrictiveness wards in 1964. Mapperley had no patients in high-restrictiveness wards in 1960 or in 1964 but the number in low-restrictiveness wards increased markedly. The position at Severalls improved somewhat, but 24 out of 41 patients were still living in highly restrictive wards in 1964. This result should be contrasted with the improvement on the other social variables described earlier.

CLINICAL CHANGES IN PATIENTS IN THE THREE HOSPITALS, 1960–1964

There was a marked improvement in clinical condition in patients at all three hospitals, between 1960 and 1964, if overall clinical category is used as a criterion. The figures are given in Tables 7.9 and 7.10 (pp. 230 and 231) and show much less difference between hospitals in 1964 than in 1960.

The mean social withdrawal scores were calculated for the three 'clinical improvement groups' separately, at each hospital, in order to determine whether group I (containing patients who were seriously ill in 1960 but who improved by at least one clinical category in 1964) improved significantly in behaviour compared with group NC (containing equivalent patients who did not improve in clinical category). The data are presented in Table 7.11 (p. 231). At Netherne and Severalls there is a highly significant decrease in social withdrawal score in group I patients compared with group NC. At

Mapperley, however, there is a significant decrease in mean score in both groups I and NC, and the decrease in group I is not much greater than that in group NC. Another interesting finding is that group M patients at Severalls (those who were moderately ill both in 1960 and in 1964) actually became *more* socially withdrawn. (This finding will be discussed in the second part of this chapter.)

It was shown in Chapter 5 that social withdrawal was highest among Netherne patients who had been in hospital more than twenty years, while at Mapperley those with more than ten years' stay also had high scores, and Severalls patients tended to be withdrawn even in the lowest length-of-stay group. It was suggested that social improvements made most initial impact on patients who had been in hospital for relatively shorter periods of time. If so, it would be expected that withdrawal scores would be decreased most among the short-stay group at Severalls, the medium-stay group at Mapperley and the long-stay group at Netherne. Figure 7.12 (p. 232) shows that this is approximately what did occur, though the improvement in the shortest-stay group at Severalls was not quite up to expectation, owing to an increase in social withdrawal in some moderately-ill patients.

Mean scores representing socially embarrassing behaviour changed very little between 1960 and 1964 at Netherne (1·2, 1·1) and Severalls (1·5, 1·3) but decreased significantly at Mapperley (2·4, 1·3). Thus there was no difference between the hospitals in 1964, according to this measure.

The change in ratings on individual items making up the S.W. and S.E. scores is shown in Tables 7.13 and 7.14 (pp. 233 and 234). It can be seen that very few patients were incontinent in 1964 (11 per cent at Severalls was the highest proportion). Violent behaviour was also extremely uncommon during the survey week in 1964.

The amount of phenothiazine drugs prescribed for patients (estimated as described in Chapter 2) changed very little at Netherne (2·2, 2·8) and Severalls (1·5, 2·3), but at Mapperley, where it was already high in 1960, the doses prescribed increased still further (3·4, 4·8). There was no evidence that changes in the dose or type of phenothiazines administered were related to any of the changes described earlier, whether clinical or social (see below for more detailed consideration of changes in drug treatment).

TIME SPENT DOING NOTHING, AND CLINICAL IMPROVEMENT
CATEGORY, 1960–1964

Since the amount of time spent doing nothing was found, in Chapter 6, to be so important in accounting for the clinical condition of the patient, analyses of variance were made of the mean changes on this variable shown by the patients in the three clinical improvement categories, separately for each hospital. The mean scores are presented in Table 7.15 (p. 234). There is a significant 'groups by occasions' interaction in each case, and the decrease in amount of time doing nothing (which looks negligible from the overall figures at Netherne and Mapperley) is found to occur almost exclusively in the group of patients who showed severe symptoms in 1960 but were found to be improved in 1964.

CHANGES IN ATTITUDE TO DISCHARGE, 1960 AND 1964

The relationship between attitude to discharge and length of stay remains very strong in each hospital taken separately, in 1964 as in 1960. There are very few differences between hospitals in the extent to which attitudes changed between 1960 and 1964.

The process of change, 1960–1968

The changes discussed so far in this chapter might have occurred at any time between 1960 and 1964. In view of the possible explanation that patients tend to improve with 'time alone' and that the social improvements merely take advantage of this fact, rather than causing the clinical improvements, it is of considerable importance to examine in more detail the changes that occur with time. Additional material is available from the full surveys carried out in 1962 at Mapperley and Severalls, and from the lesser surveys of all three hospitals made in January 1968. The latter material does not include any personal interviews by the investigators but only the ward behaviour scales, the occupation and outside-contact inventories, and a schedule of nurses' attitudes which contained the same items as had been used by the sociologist in earlier surveys. The 1968 information was collected about 7½ years after the 1960 material. For Severalls patients the follow-up period was 7 years 9 months, for Netherne patients 7 years 6 months and for Mapperley patients 7 years 4 months.

These discrepancies do not affect the interpretation of the findings. The scores allow examination of the changes over time in more detail.

OUTCOME IN JANUARY 1968

Table 7.16 (p. 235) shows the 7½-year outcome of patients who were interviewed in 1960.

Twenty-five patients died. There was a non-significant excess of deaths among patients with marked poverty of speech or muteness in 1960. The deaths of several patients were probably due indirectly to their mental condition. One patient was found dead in a nearby lake. One catatonic patient died of subacute obstruction following years of faecal retention. One patient died from drowning after falling in her bath (she weighed over 16 stone) and another grossly obese patient (over 17 stone) died of broncho-pneumonia. Three other patients died of pneumonia and two of diabetes. None of the other causes of death appeared to be related, even indirectly, to the patient's psychiatric state or to circumstances of life connected with it.

Eight patients at Netherne were living in hospital but working outside, and eight at Mapperley were living in hospital-supervised hostels outside but attending the wards daily—these sixteen have been included with the in-patients in January 1968, since information was available about them. Four patients were transferred to other hospitals.

Fifty-three patients had been discharged and were still out of the parent hospital in January 1968. Several had been discharged and re-admitted and re-discharged (one had been discharged six times). Characteristics which differentiated the 53 discharged patients from the rest are shown in Table 7.17 (p. 235).

Clinical and social factors measured in 1960 acted as good predictors of which patients would be discharged early. Of the 26 patients discharged by 1964, 19 (73 per cent) were only moderately impaired in 1960 and 21 (81 per cent) had then wanted to leave.

The patients discharged after 1964 were more disabled in 1960 and did not have such favourable attitudes at that time. Out of 27 patients, 14 had severe speech symptoms and 13 had moderate symptoms, in 1960. Table 7.18 (p. 236) shows that 12 out of the 14 discharged patients who had severe symptoms in 1960 had improved by 1964, that is, they were members of group I, while only two were members of group NC. This association is very highly significant and suggests that clinical improvement is likely to help towards the patient's discharge.

PATIENTS STILL IN HOSPITAL IN JANUARY 1968

The purpose of this section is not so much to compare the level of functioning of patients at the three hospitals as to consider how the level changed, at each hospital, on the four occasions of testing. However, it should be pointed out that Mapperley still had a small excess (12 per cent more than Netherne) of patients who had been in hospital more than twenty years in 1960, although this does not reach statistical significance. All the conclusions have therefore been checked to see whether they apply when only the shorter-stay patients (who are automatically matched for age) are considered at the three hospitals. In fact, no modification is required to the discussion. Tables 7.19 and 7.20 (pp. 236 and 237) give the distribution of the remaining 191 patients in terms of age and length of stay in 1960. The rest of the analysis in this section is based on these 191 patients only.

The mean scores on social withdrawal, favourable nurses' attitudes, and occupation, for 191 patients rated in 1960, 1962, 1964 and 1968, are shown in Figure 7.21 (p. 237).

The addition of data collected in 1962 and 1968 considerably modifies the picture presented earlier in this chapter. All the improvements previously described were well under way by 1962 at both Mapperley and Severalls but, while Severalls continued to progress after this year (though at a slower rate), there was a decline at Mapperley and much of the improvement had been lost by the beginning of 1968. There was no survey at Netherne in 1962 so that the turning point cannot be dated exactly but, again, the improvements registered between 1960 and 1964 had mostly been lost by the beginning of 1968. The social environment of Netherne retained its advantages compared with the other two hospitals, however, and the social withdrawal of its patients remained less.

Figure 7.21 also shows a strikingly parallel development of clinical and social changes at each hospital. Improvement in the social measures is accompanied by a decrease in mean social withdrawal score, and when the social environment reverts to the previous level, there is a concomitant increase in social withdrawal.

The largest deterioration in social withdrawal was at Mapperley between 1962 (when the mean score was least) and 1968 (when it was almost as high as in 1960). Table 7.23 (p. 240) shows the distribution of change in social withdrawal score and occupation score between these two occasions of measurement. Splitting two ways as close to the median as possible, the relationship is highly significant. Twenty patients out of 55 show a deterioration of two points or more in both social withdrawal and occupation score. The correlation between the mean changes in score on the two variables is 0·27 (p < 0·05).

Mean scores on four variables are shown, separately for three length-of-stay groups, in Figure 7.22 (pp. 238-9). It is clear that length of stay (and age, which is also controlled) does not account for any of the differences between the hospitals. Indeed, the over-21-year group at Severalls is socially as well off in 1968 as the equivalent group at Netherne—a really remarkable improvement—and the difference in mean S.W. score is lowest in this group. It appears that, apart from the shortest-stay group, the improvement at Severalls had not reached its peak though it was levelling off. The mean S.W. score seemed likely to decrease further at Severalls.

Thirty-seven patients were still 45 years of age or younger in January 1968. Their mean social withdrawal scores are compared with those of older patients in Figure 7.24 (p. 241), and do not indicate a more favourable course of events. In fact, at Severalls, the younger patients do not even share the general improvement between 1964 and 1968.

DETERIORATION OF PATIENTS WITH MODERATE CLINICAL IMPAIRMENT IN 1960

Patients who showed no, or only moderate, impairment in 1960 (members of clinical subgroups 1*a* and 1*b*) are compared on the mean S.W. score with more severely impaired patients in Figure 7.25 (p. 241). At Netherne and Mapperley the two groups, while remaining significantly different, show a similar pattern of change over the years. At Severalls there is a striking convergence of scores, and the small group of nine patients who were only moderately impaired in 1960 . increased in mean S.W. score from 1·4 to 4·8.

This increase of social withdrawal among the least handicapped patients at Severalls runs counter to the strong overall trend for patients to improve. This may relate to the way the wards were reorganised. In 1960, there had been an association between mental state and ward organisation—the more handicapped the patient the more restrictive his ward tended to be (Figure 7.26, p. 242). (This relationship also held at the other two hospitals.) This could have been brought about either by those living in restrictive wards becoming more withdrawn after arriving on the ward, or by the more handicapped being sent to live on such wards. Both processes may well have been at work. After 1960 there was a major organisational change: the care of the non-geriatric patients, including new admissions, was divided among five 'firms' under separate consultant psychiatrists. Each firm had only a handful of wards for the care of its patients. In an effort to ensure that they had an equal number of the most handicapped, long-stay patients were randomly allocated to the firms, and by 1962 the association between mental state and ward organisation had disappeared. The more handicapped were no longer living on the more restricted wards (Figure 7.26). There had also been a dramatic drop in the restrictiveness of the wards but by 1964 the situation had changed again. There was still no relation between mental state and ward organisation, but the restrictiveness of the wards had increased markedly (Figure 7.26). It is possible that the care of patients with a wide range of handicap on the same ward had forced the nursing staff to allow less freedom. Whatever the reason, the changes meant that those least handicapped in 1960 at Severalls were living on considerably more restrictive wards in 1964 than 1960 or 1962.

We have already noted in Chapter 4 (see Figure 4.3, p. 201) evidence that the ward can have an influence on social withdrawal irrespective of the time patients spend unoccupied, and Figure 7.27 (p. 243) illustrates this in more detail. In all survey years social withdrawal tends to be greater in the more restrictive wards, even when the amount of time spent unoccupied by each patient is allowed for. What happened at Severalls after 1960 suggests that changes in the ward organisation can lead to changes both in social withdrawal and in clinical category.

We have seen that the reorganisation of the wards at Severalls meant that the least handicapped patients spent a good deal more time under more restrictive conditions, but it is not clear just how this led to increased social withdrawal. Ten of the moderately handicapped patients were more socially withdrawn by 1964 (although none deteriorated in mental state). But, since only three of these ten showed a large increase in time unoccupied, it appears that way of life on the ward can influence social withdrawal without any effect on the time spent in employment or leisure activities. This might well be the start of a lengthy process which proceeds through major increases in unoccupied time to culminate in a deterioration in mental state. The effect of changes in ward organisation on *both* social withdrawal and mental state is most clearly demonstrated from material at Severalls, although the numbers involved are too small to make the result more than suggestive. Table 7.28(*a*), on p. 244, shows that patients stood most chance of improving in mental state between 1960 and 1964 if both the amount of time spent unoccupied and the restrictiveness of their ward were reduced (proportion improved 0·90), less chance if only time spent unoccupied was reduced (0·64), and still less chance if only the restrictiveness of the ward improved (0·35) or neither changed (0·14). Table 7.28(*b*) shows a similar trend for social withdrawal. Both results suggest that time spent unoccupied and restrictiveness of the ward have independent effects on the patients, although a reduction in time spent unoccupied is the more influential in reducing handicap. The way patients were re-allocated to wards at Severalls after 1960, and the fact that the association between ward organisation and mental state disappeared, makes it unlikely that the apparent effect of the ward is explained by patients first improving and then being sent to less restrictive wards.

In 1960, the size of the ward was strongly related to the amount of restrictiveness, at all the three hospitals ($r = +0.869$, $N = 20$, $p < 0.001$). In 1964, however, there was very little association ($r = +0.337$, $N = 15$, $p > 0.1$).

PHENOTHIAZINE TREATMENT

Although there has been no evidence in the analysis so far presented that changes in phenothiazine medication were responsible for clinical improvement, it is important to consider this matter in more detail. The surveys at Mapperley and Severalls in 1960 and 1962 provide an opportunity, since there was considerable clinical change during this period. E.C.T. was rarely used at the time of any survey and there was no change in the amount and type of night-time sedation. The relationship between change in drug administration and clinical improvement is set out in Table 7.29 (p. 245).

Only 19 out of 112 patients received no phenothiazines at all during the two years, and only 5 stopped treatment. Forty-five patients remained on exactly the same medication. In 29 cases, there were minor changes of dose (for example, an increase from 375 mg. to 450 mg. of Chlorpromazine) or type of drug (for example, a change from Chlorpromazine 150 mg. to Thioridazine 150 mg.). In 34 cases, there were major changes of dose (for example, from $37\frac{1}{2}$ mg. to 75 mg. of Prochlorperazine) or from one to another type of phenothiazine (for example, from 150 mg. Chlorpromazine to 60 mg. Trifluoperazine). Twenty-five patients were receiving phenothiazine in 1962 but not in 1960.

There is no evidence that change in drug treatment was responsible in any way for the clinical improvement.

The final discussion of this material will be held over to Chapter 10, following a descriptive account of certain wards and patients (which make the meaning of the quantitative data easier to appreciate), and the presentation of results from a comparable survey in an American County Hospital which, although very preliminary and tentative, also provides some interesting ideas about the organisation of mental hospitals.

Summary

1. The greatest social improvements between 1960 and 1964 took place at Severalls Hospital, where the environment experienced by patients in the series became little different to that at Mapperley. Netherne still retained an overall superiority.

2. Although there was a very highly significant improvement on all five social measures of the individual Severalls patient's social environment (e.g. outside contact, nurses' attitudes, etc.) there was still a substantial proportion living in highly restrictive wards.

3. The clinical condition, measured by interview ratings, of patients at all three hospitals improved between 1960 and 1964.

Social withdrawal actually increased, however, in certain patients at Severalls who were only moderately impaired.

4. Patients who spent less time 'doing nothing' in 1964 were, on the whole, the patients whose clinical condition improved. There was a very highly significant interaction.

5. By January 1968, 19 per cent of patients were discharged and still out of hospital, 9 per cent had died, and 64 per cent were still in-patients. If the 3 per cent of day patients and the 3 per cent of night patients are taken into account, there was little difference between the hospitals. Clinical and social factors measured in 1960 acted as good predictors of which patients would be discharged relatively early. Patients who improved in clinical condition between 1960 and 1964 had a significantly better chance of being discharged during the subsequent four years.

6. The progress of patients in the three hospitals was compared using one clinical factor (social withdrawal) and three social factors (nurses' attitudes, occupation and outside contact) measured in 1960, 1962 (except at Netherne), 1964 and 1968. Most improvement took place between 1960 and 1962. Thereafter the rate of improvement fell off and, at Mapperley and Netherne, was actually reversed. Some improvement was still taking place at Severalls between 1964 and 1968 and seemed likely to continue for a time.

7. Improvement of the social environment of a hospital was always accompanied by a decrease in social withdrawal in the patients there. Clinical and social deterioration also always occurred together.

8. A detailed analysis of phenothiazine medication at Mapperley and Severalls hospitals between 1960 and 1962 when clinical improvement was greatest, yielded no evidence that changes in drug treatment, the addition of another drug, or beginning drug treatment, were in any way responsible.

8

THE NUMERICAL DATA
ILLUSTRATED BY A DESCRIPTIVE
ACCOUNT OF SELECTED WARDS
AND REPRESENTATIVE PATIENTS

Practically all the material in this book is presented in numerical form. Such indices stand for real and important characteristics of personal condition and social environment, and we would reject the suggestion that is sometimes made (fortunately rather rarely) that they are meaningless abstractions. We have deliberately chosen to make our investigation in this way because we do not think that the most animated and evocative description by the most perceptive participant observers could possibly answer the questions we set ourselves. We do not, of course, discount their value, but they have another purpose and are complementary to the present approach.

In this chapter we shall try to give life to some of our figures and to illustrate some of the processes they measure, by means of an account of three particular wards. Two of them cater for severely-handicapped patients, but they represented different stages in the progress from the old-fashioned kindly but deadening 'back' ward to the modern 'therapeutic community'. There was no ward in any of the three hospitals which was equivalent to that described by L. Wing (1956) and Folkard (1956)—where gallons of paraldehyde were dispensed weekly and the 'padded room' still existed as a possible means of seclusion. Our three hospitals, in 1960, were even farther away, of course, from the days when physical means of restraint, such as anklets, straps or strait-jackets, were used. Such techniques have fortunately been less common in British hospitals than elsewhere, but were never really necessary, as Conolly pointed out over a hundred years ago (1856).

Nevertheless, Kerry Ward and Longfield Villa do allow a comparison between the old and the new. The comparison is unfair and unscientific—that is the problem with descriptive work. Kerry Ward may well have started out with more difficult patients than Longfield, whereas the impression an observer received from visiting the two wards one after the other was undoubtedly that, in part at any rate, they were each responsible, for better or for worse, for the clinical condition of their patients. We undertook this investigation in order to try to reach an answer to this kind of question, and the results presented in earlier chapters do, we think, go a long way towards answering it. We must emphasise, however, that our conclusions do not rest upon the kind of 'evidence' presented in this chapter.

We should also like to point out that the sisters-in-charge and the nurses on both wards were pleasant, kindly, sympathetic people, who gave us every facility we needed for observation and spoke with complete frankness about their problems. They represented the nursing traditions they were brought up in and their different attitudes in no way reflected systematic differences in personality.

Twenty-two of the patients we studied were living in Kerry Ward, and twelve in Longfield Villa, in 1960. Very brief notes are appended about six patients from each ward, chosen because they seemed to be roughly equivalent in length of stay and condition on admission, and in underlying handicap at the time of interview. Sixteen patients were living in Downswood Villa in 1960 and brief notes are given about six of them. The function of this villa was to provide a fairly normal environment for long-stay patients who might be discharged from hospital within a reasonable space of time.

Kerry Ward

In 1960, Kerry Ward had the highest restrictiveness score of all the wards we studied. It contained almost one hundred women, mainly diagnosed as schizophrenic, all of whom had been in hospital at least one year. The median length of stay was fourteen years and one-third had lived in the hospital continuously for over twenty years. Thirty-eight per cent were over 60 years of age. The average age was 56 with a range from 30 to 81 years. The ward itself had a large living area with three main dormitories. One dormitory was reserved for 46 'defective' patients and another for the 'better' patients. There was also a fourth small dormitory for 'sick' patients. At the time of the survey most of the 7 sick patients had minor complaints. Patients with 'heavy colds' were put into bed for several days—'it is not a nice job wiping their noses'. There were seven side-rooms—two were for the two most active ward-workers among the patients and the other five for the seriously disturbed, one of whom spent most of her time in bed. There was no padded room in the ward.

Six staff were usually on duty at a time between 7 a.m. and 8.30 p.m., working in two shifts. Most had little experience of the ward—only three of the eleven nurses had worked there as long as six months. The sister-in-charge, however, had been there two years.

The ward was on the first floor of the main hospital building with no ready access to the grounds. Its door was always locked. Practically the whole of the patients' lives was spent within the ward. There was little contact with the rest of the hospital and practically none with the world outside. No patient went home and only a couple visited the local town. Less than half were visited by relatives, and those not all regularly. Visiting rules had recently been liberalised but the patients were not aware of this and, in effect, the old visiting hours were still adhered to.

The hospital had extensive and attractive grounds, a hospital shop and a cinema; and there was work available for some patients about the hospital—either in the grounds, in the laundry or doing domestic work on the wards. But on Kerry Ward only five patients were allowed to leave without the supervision of a nurse, and only one worked elsewhere in the hospital (part-time work in the laundry). Nurses took groups of patients for walks but these were irregular and brief and at the time of the survey no outing had taken place for some time.

Movement about the ward itself was also restricted. Store rooms were locked ('to keep them tidy') and washrooms except at meal-times. The dormitories were locked during the day to prevent patients going to bed too early. Other activities such as bathing were subject to close control. The bathroom was locked and no one used it except when supervised on 'bathdays'. On these occasions, a nurse and five patients helped with undressing and dressing. A senior nurse was always present—not only to help but to watch out for bruises, rashes and injuries. Each patient had her hair washed as a matter of course once a week during bathing: 'it's difficult when they are in clothes'. There were no exceptions.

Such practices are, of course, not uncommon in 'total institutions'. Goffman has drawn attention to the stripping process by which many of the characteristics which differentiate individuals are removed. The process continues over the years; skills are neglected, overfamiliar or even impolite terms of address are used, conventional greetings are ignored and so on. These deprivations can be resisted for a time by the richness of the social skills and equipment the inmate brings with him. Our patients were well beyond the initial stage of stripping and their social poverty can be measured most clearly by their lack of possessions: most of the things brought in at the time of admission had worn out years before and there was little they could call their own. Very few patients even owned a toothbrush—teeth were cleaned, if at all, with the aid of a piece of lint. Almost all clothing was provided by the hospital but it was not regarded as the patient's own. At times a patient might receive the same dress back from the laundry but this depended on some chance recognition by the nurse giving out clothing. Most was handed out as it came, according to rough size. The same was true of the overcoats handed round when parties of patients went out for walks. Storage space was in any case scarce. Two patients had wardrobes in their rooms but all other private clothing was kept in a locked store room. The only other storage space was provided by eighteen small lockers. Personal possessions were not to be seen about the ward: 'they get stolen and I tell them to put anything away'. There was, in fact, little that could have been displayed. A detailed count of possessions was made for the 22 patients in the series who were living in the ward. Twelve possessed nothing at all: 5 owned one or two items (a kilt; a cardigan and apron; a dress and pair of shoes; a cardigan; beads). Only 5 of the the 22 patients possessed much else of significance and two of these hardly used their things, which were kept in the store room. Few of the women had any effective control of the 'front' they presented to the world. Mirrors, cosmetics and ornaments were lacking: and even the primitive control provided by a comb was largely absent. Most patients had their hair combed each morning by one of the nurses, and that had to last all day. Although many patients were overweight, no one had foundation garments.

These deficiencies are easily measured and appreciated. It is less easy to assess the significance of the lack of privacy on the ward, which was almost total. The two working patients with side-rooms were the only people with any opportunity to be alone. Baths were unscreened and the lavatory doors unlockable.

The general drabness of life was evident in the lack of photographs, ornaments, postcards, pictures and reminders of other worlds. This poverty was continued in the decor—mainly browns and buffs with little brightness or pattern. Patients never used the washrooms for washing clothes; no patient used the kitchen; there were no mirrors in the dormitories. There were three daily papers and four weekly magazines but few patients saw them. On the other hand, the television set seemed to be perpetually on.

In all these matters patients were treated alike. Nevertheless, patients could be *perceived* by the staff as individuals. The three nurses who had been on the ward for more than a few months had no difficulty in giving detailed accounts of each woman; often knowing, for example, exactly where she was to be found at any time during the day. The others could not do this, and the transfer of nurses from ward to ward at short intervals added to the process of stripping.

An outstanding feature of ward life was the degree to which patients were caught up in a routine geared to the economic requirements of the ward. Throughout the day, groups of patients were treated in a similar fashion: most were in bed by eight o'clock, eighty queued to have their hair combed each morning and forty were taken to the lavatory at set times during the day. But as these figures demonstrate, differences were recognised. Only the most incontinent, for example, were got up at set times during the night. Nor had the labelling led to consistent groupings of patients. The two allowed to control the television set had their hair washed during the weekly bath like everybody else. A grouping formed in relation to one activity was usually ignored in another.

On the whole, the practice of personal skills was not encouraged. There was considerable pressure for patients to feed themselves, but many more could clearly have combed their own hair. Competence in a few essential activities such as eating and use of the lavatory was required for the smooth running of the ward but very little else was deemed necessary. All beds, for example, were made for the patients and there was no evidence that the staff were dissatisfied with this arrangement. Some patients helped with ward work but, with the staff largely occupied in domestic chores, help from a handful of patients was quite sufficient. Without moving nurses away from this work there was little chance of the ward system itself generating pressure to develop or maintain individual skills. The only pressure came from outside the ward. Two occupational therapists visited the ward on most days of the week and managed to occupy some of the patients, though their achievements were modest.

It is difficult to explain all that we saw in terms of the exigencies of caring for a large number of patients. Some practices seemed no more than a self-imposed search for order on the part of the staff. Reasons were readily given for what went on: the patients did not use the kitchen because of the risk of spreading dysentery and the ward was locked because of the few 'escapers'.

That the pursuit of order went beyond practical requirements is not surprising. Standards in such circumstances easily become ends in themselves and are easily imposed. There was, however, little sign of the 'tyrannisation' which Goffman has described as flourishing under such conditions. Inmates can be subjected to a series of highly detailed and petty regulations—prisoners, for example, may be dressed to numbers shouted out by a guard. There was no sign of such elaboration on this ward, although patients had to ask permission to do things that obviously cut across the main activities of the ward—to get clothes from the store room, to light a cigarette, to leave the ward, and so on. But the ward is better characterised by the poverty of rules, which were few and simple, fitting the tedium of the daily round.

The day began early. No one was allowed up before 6.45 a.m.: but by the time the night nurse went round pulling bed clothes off most were up and about. This nurse had already started the task of washing by the time the day staff arrived about 7 a.m. Two nurses supervised washing. Twenty patients were completely washed, dressed and helped to use the lavatory and a further thirty were washed—face, neck and hands—and 'tidied'. Fifteen used the basin-room at a time—some washing and others drying. Each had fresh water but the use of individual flannels and towels had been introduced only the previous week. After washing, most queued outside the washroom for their hair to be combed—since hair was cut short this took only a few seconds.

The main living area of the ward was opened about 7.30 a.m.—after some of the better patients had laid the breakfast table. Patients came through from washing and sat at their own places (all but twelve knew where to sit). The meal began about eight o'clock. The organisation of meal-times was worked out so that the various types of feeding-problem could be supervised by the small number of staff. The table for 'co-operative' patients was closest to the serving-hatch —these patients pointed out to sister which others were not eating, and helped with serving. Strategically placed at a distance from the serving-hatch was a table for the 'over-eaters', who were not allowed to collect their own food but were waited upon. In the centre of the room were two small tables, one for patients who had to be hand fed, the other for those who needed close supervision. Another table nearby was for patients who needed urging to eat. Most of the nurses were concentrated around these three tables. At the top of the room was an elite table for workers.

The staff brought food to the 'special' tables, and selected patients collected food for the others. Tea, which had had milk and sugar added, was served at each of the tables in jugs. Most of the food (such as bacon) came from the main kitchen; but the bread, although cut there, was buttered on the ward on the previous afternoon. After the meal, all waited until 'sedatives' had been given out. Grace was said by the nurse in charge at about 8.45 a.m. By then most patients had sat at the table for over an hour. After grace, forty were led off as a group to the lavatory and washroom. During the next hour the main living area was tidied and, while this was being done by nurses and a few 'workers', sixty patients were locked in a small corridor outside. On the first day of our visit we had to push our way through these patients to get to the sister's office. No one was able to leave the corridor during this time.

Once back on the ward the majority sat about doing nothing, although on most mornings the two visiting occupational therapists managed to keep twenty or so occupied at knitting, needlework or basket-making. By midday preparation for the second meal was under way. Forty were again taken to the lavatory. The meal took again over an hour, not ending until sedatives had been given out: 'We have to hand out the medicine while they are all together, as they would be clearing off all round the ward. I can do it in fifteen minutes then; otherwise it would take an hour.' While the same forty patients were taken to the washroom the ward was swept. The only activity in the afternoon was provided by the two occupational therapists who, for an hour, managed to get nearly half the ward joining in dancing, singing and 'free movement'. Tea took less time: it began at four o'clock and lasted about half an hour, and was associated with the same toileting procedures. Then until supper at 7.30 p.m. patients were left to their own devices. Some watched television, more sat near the two fires doing nothing; a few knitted or read. The staff were all engaged on some domestic or medical duty and were not seen talking or mixing with the patients. Supper was a relatively short affair, and by eight o'clock things were well under way to get the ward to bed. Within half an hour of supper the staff with the help of five patients had got most patients into bed with their clothes rolled up in a bundle under each bed. The nurse left on the ward was helped, if necessary, by a night sister who passed through the ward every hour. On three occasions during the night fifteen from the largest dormitory were raised and taken to the lavatory. However, by 9.30 p.m. the whole ward was relatively quiet: all sedatives had been given out, the fifteen patients had been raised for the first time by the night nurse and the lights in the 'best' dormitory were turned out. Only two or three remained up to watch television.

This was the daily cycle. Each day was very much the same except that at weekends the occupational therapists were absent.

In spite of the large amount of control by the staff over what went on, there were long periods when most patients were simply waiting for the next stage of the cycle to begin: this waiting was mostly spent in apathetic inactivity, in doing absolutely nothing. All but one of the twenty-two patients in the series spent three hours a day sitting at a meal table, and half were totally unoccupied except when eating or at toilet. Only seven made any attempt to occupy themselves when left alone, usually by looking at television. Some did odd jobs about the ward—but the reward bore no relationship to outside standards. One patient who worked extremely well for seven hours a day was given only four shillings a week. There was in fact little evidence of a system of reward or punishment and the staff saw no need for one. Questioning about such matters was met by puzzlement. We did note a nurse shouting at a patient across the length of the ward, 'Flossie, come off the radiator'. She explained that the patient tended to get chilblains. A few patients had rooms of their own but we could gather no suggestion by staff or patients that these were seen as privileges to be withdrawn for misconduct. Longer acquaintance might well have revealed some reflection of the elaborate system of reward and punishment described by Belknap in an American mental hospital, but our overall impression was that it was of little moment for the running of this ward.

The staff were generally pessimistic about the patients. The sister in charge thought only one of the twenty-two patients in the series could do useful work for the hospital (she was the worker receiving four shillings a week); and a nurse who knew them well thought two patients could do so. About the same number were thought to be able to appreciate the value of money or visit the local shops alone. Some opinions did, however, run counter to current practice. The sister thought six patients should be encouraged to have their own clothing and the nurse thought that as many as half the patients should. Only one was felt to need to be on a locked ward, and the sister felt that six patients (the nurse thought only one) could be allowed to bath alone. Both agreed that the 'workers' should receive more—the sister thought the one already mentioned should get 7s. 6d. and the nurse considered 10s. would be appropriate. But on the whole they believed that the hospital provided for the patients' wants. They both mentioned that many loved fragrant soap (from the shop) and the nurse thought shampoos, talcum powder and toothpaste would be widely appreciated. On the whole the nurses accepted the current system. The sister looked forward only to an improvement in the domestic equipment of the ward—a better kitchen, a refrigerator, and so on.

By the time of our visit in 1962 the ward had been closed, and extensive alterations were being carried out, including its division into separate units. On a subsequent visit its partitions, new flooring, bright curtains and flowers and colourful paintwork made it difficult to follow the topography of the old ward. Most of the patients had been moved to different wards. Of the original twenty-two in the series, one had been transferred to another hospital—her condition had not improved. One mute chronic catatonic patient had died from intestinal obstruction following years of faecal retention. Two patients had been discharged (both had expressed some desire to leave when interviewed in 1960). One had been markedly incoherent when seen in 1960; the other showed marked poverty of affect and speech, but the case-notes suggested that both had improved considerably before discharge. Five of the other eighteen had improved by 1962, and eight by 1964. Attitudes to discharge crystallised somewhat: by 1964 only six instead of thirteen were indifferent or mute, seven instead of three wanted to leave, and five instead of two wanted to stay.

The social environment of the eighteen patients at the time of the 1962 survey had definitely improved. Half of them had left the ward on the day of the survey, for example, compared with only one in 1960. However, the restrictiveness of the regime to which the eighteen patients were exposed, although it was markedly reduced from 88 per cent in 1960 to 44 per cent in 1962, climbed again to 70 per cent in 1964 (the 1962 and 1964 figures represent the average of several different wards).

Certain indices showed a more continuous improvement. For example, the average number of personal possessions owned by the eighteen patients rose from 2·1 in 1960 to 8·8 in 1962 and 16·6 in 1964. While only one patient owned her own comb in 1960, eight did so in 1962 and seventeen in 1964. The nurses became increasingly optimistic in their attitudes, giving an average of 3·3, 4·6 and 6·1 positive opinions on the three survey days. However, the reduction in amount of time spent doing nothing was levelling off by 1964: it was 7 hours 5 minutes in 1960, 5 hours 1 minute in 1962 and 4 hours 23 minutes in 1964. The reduction was largely due to more time being spent at occupational therapy. There had been a slight increase in leisure activity (from 1 hour 6 minutes in 1960 to 1 hour 39 minutes in 1962) but almost all this time (92 per cent) was spent watching television.

SIX PATIENTS IN KERRY WARD

Kerry patient No. 6. Mrs Veronica A

Mrs A had been admitted to hospital in 1945 at the age of 25. She thought she was God in the Spirit and that she was being poisoned. She laughed to herself and stared vacantly about her in the street. She was dirty, unkempt, violent, and said on admission that she wanted to be killed. Thereafter she was noted to mutter incoherently to herself, to listen and reply to voices, and later became totally mute apart from laughing and talking to herself. She was doubly incontinent. She was divorced while in hospital.

At interview in 1960 she spoke only a few words in answer to questions, but these were relevant and understandable. She sat looking fixedly in front of her, with a dejected expression, hands folded in her lap and clasping a worn handbag (clinical group 4).[1] Her hair was awry and cut short, and a leucotomy scar was visible. She had no make-up but her clothes were fairly neat. She was quite indifferent about leaving hospital. She knew how much a postage stamp cost and the name of the Queen.

In 1962 she spoke rather more but still had marked poverty of affect and speech, with an expressionless face and quiet manner (clinical group 4). The only three notes made in the case-records between the two surveys made reference to her institutionalised appearance, lethargy and lack of spontaneous talk.

In 1964, Mrs A spoke considerably more, occasionally making a spontaneous remark, and showed less flattening of affect (clinical group 1 *b*). She said that, although she didn't mind staying in hospital she would rather leave and work in a factory. She had once visited her mother at home and was fairly well informed about events in the world outside hospital. Her appearance was smart, her hair well done and her lipstick applied carefully. The charge nurse said that her visit home had not been successful because she was three hours dressing herself and hardly spoke. The impression was of considerable improvement, however.

Kerry patient No. 9. Miss Cissie B

Miss B was first admitted in 1933 when she was 25. She was then mute, stood motionless in one position and showed flexibilitas cerea. The case-records indicated no change in her condition and the most recent note stated that she was indifferent, mute, vacant and resistive, that she was incontinent and had to be hand-fed.

At interview in 1960 she did not say a word, but sat in her chair with a dejected expression, with her head on her chest, making tiny noises which gradually changed into open muttering and then died

---

[1] The clinical groups are described in Chapter 2.

away again into small movements of the lips and face (clinical group 5). She occasionally made involuntary movements of the arms. Her dress was hospital issue, her hair had the usual 'pudding basin' cut and she wore no make-up.

In 1962, Miss B was still mute. She held her hands clasped in front of her chest, rubbing the fingers together. She made continuous mouth movements, chewing, sucking and so on, with small unintelligible sounds (clinical group 5). She was not wearing her false teeth. The case-notes indicated that this was her usual condition.

In 1964 there was no change (clinical group 5). She had undergone resection for a large bowel carcinoma but was physically well at the time of interview.

Kerry patient No. 11. Mrs Flossie C

Mrs C was admitted in 1935 at the age of 31. She was at that time restless, incontinent and mute, and refused food. Later she spoke only rarely in a high-pitched babyish voice, frequently giggled to herself and became very obese. There had been some improvement in recent years. She helped in the ward kitchen, with ward cleaning, and could make some conversation.

At interview she showed very marked flattening of affect but made a few remarks indicating that she wanted to stay in hospital (clinical group 4). Her dress was untidy and dirty and her hair cut very short. She had no make-up. She had no knowledge about the outside world and could not say how much a postage stamp cost.

In 1962 she was slightly more in contact during the interview and still wanted to stay in hospital (clinical group 4). Her appearance was rather neater but her hairstyle remained as before.

In 1964 there was little change (clinical group 4).

Kerry patient No. 14. Miss Frances D

Miss D was admitted to hospital in 1930 at the age of 23. She thought that people talked about her and said she was going to have a baby. She said her food was poisoned. In hospital, she became solitary, impulsively aggressive, and spoke irrationally and incoherently. She was noisy in response to auditory hallucinations.

At interview she had a markedly flat affect and, although she spoke fairly freely, there was very little content to what she said (clinical group 4). When asked how she liked being in hospital she said, 'It's all right. I'm getting used to it now.' She thought a postage stamp cost 2*d*. and greatly underestimated the cost of a journey to her own home. She did not know the Queen's name. Her hair was cut in the same 'pudding basin' style as the other patients and she had no make-up. Her clothes were ordinary hospital issue.

According to the case-notes she improved after this, went out once a week with her sister and seemed very sensible in her conversation. Her sister agreed to take her home for a trial period, which was a success, and so she was discharged at the beginning of 1961. When she was followed up at the time of the second survey she was still reasonably well, keeping house for her sister.

Kerry patient No. 18. Miss Karen E

Miss E was admitted in 1948 at the age of 33. She had lost interest in everything, became untidy and dirty and almost mute, and had visions of crosses. In hospital she was solitary and apathetic, resenting the slightest change in daily routine, had to be hand-fed and was occasionally resistive. She was receiving Taractan 60 mg. t.d.s.

At interview in 1960 she was completely mute and motionless, with blue hands and feet (clinical group 5). She had to be led everywhere and was fed by the nurses.

This condition continued until mid-1961 when she began to improve after a course of six electro-convulsive treatments followed by Chlorpromazine 100 mg. t.d.s. She began to work in the ward kitchen and the needleroom and wrote a sensible letter to her relatives. Towards the end of 1961 she began to go out for car-rides with her sister and spoke slowly but rationally on these occasions. At interview in 1962 she spoke fairly realistically (but very slowly) of her situation. 'I would like to get a job but my sister can't keep me. She's busy' (clinical group 4). She said she would like to leave, but would be content to stay if she could work in the hospital: 'My sister said she thought that they were needing patients here.' Miss E was partly informed about everyday events—she knew the price of a postage stamp but not how much it would cost to get home. She thought the Queen's name was Margaret. Her appearance was slightly idiosyncratic, with a shock of curled grey hair standing up from her head, blue-framed spectacles on the tip of her nose and a smart bright pink cardigan. She was slightly bent and would have passed as a 'little old lady' outside hospital. Her affect was still markedly flat.

In 1964 the situation was much the same. She continued to go out with her sister once a fortnight but had developed the habit of repeatedly kneeling on the floor. She did this twice during the interview, without explanation. The impression of a small bird-like woman, with a smart but slightly eccentric appearance, remained. Her conversation was still very slow (and became slower the longer the interview continued) but what she did say was to the point. Her affect was still markedly flat (clinical group 1 *c*). She no longer wished to leave hospital.

Kerry patient No. 22. Miss Jane F

Miss F was admitted to hospital in 1949 at the age of 30. She was then agitated and screaming. Voices told her dreadful and disgusting things and she thought that she and her mother were being persecuted and injured. In hospital she was solitary, standing idly about for hours at a time, occasionally shouting inexplicably, but sometimes doing a little needlework. She frequently muttered and giggled to herself and was often difficult with taking food.

At interview in 1960, her conversation was rational and to the point (clinical group 1 *b*). She thought it was a nice hospital but of course she would like to be discharged though she didn't know where to go. Her parents were dead and she had no brothers or sisters. She thought a stamp cost 2½*d*. and did not know the price of the journey home. She was familiar with the names of members of the royal family. She looked much younger than her 40 years and was demurely attractive in appearance, though her clothes were hospital issue and she wore no make-up. There were no florid symptoms but she seemed rather apathetic. It was difficult to understand why she remained in hospital—particularly in a ward like Kerry.

Between 1960 and 1962 she was considered for a job outside hospital but, although her typing was good, she completely lacked initiative. She would come into the occupational therapy department in the morning and stand until someone told her to take off her coat. Separate and specific instructions were needed for her to take up the typing paper, type a letter, put it in an envelope, put on a stamp, etc. Her shorthand speed was 70 words per minute. At interview she was timid, over-polite and looked much closer to her real age. She sat with her hands folded in her lap, head bowed, and made the same sort of conversation as on the previous occasion (clinical group 1 *b*). She no longer wanted to leave hospital.

By 1964 she had put on some weight but was attractive in appearance and wore lipstick. She had settled down in a new ward (a reconstructed portion of the old Kerry Ward). She went into town once a fortnight with a friend, worked in the nurses' teaching unit as a typist, and was quite content to stay in hospital. She had no symptoms of schizophrenia (clinical group 1 *a*).

Longfield Villa

In marked contrast to Kerry Ward, Longfield Villa had been set up in 1956 with the specific purpose in mind of 'resocialising' the most severely handicapped female schizophrenic patients. The neighbouring villa, for similarly handicapped men, was part of the same unit and all daytime activities were shared. Each nurse in the Resocialisation Unit was handed a simple statement of aims and methods. Patients who improved were transferred to another ward which was more oriented towards resettlement outside the hospital. The patients in the Unit were, on the whole, less disturbed than those in Kerry Ward, though the type of handicap was, in general, the same.

A statement published about the Unit in 1957 made the point that 'habit-training' tended to emphasise the passive dependence of patients on staff so that there was a real possibility that individuality and initiative were smothered; and argued for 'the maximum of integration of both patients and staff, in the framework of a permissive, flexible and democratic environment'. In 1956 male and female patients were moved into two adjacent villas surrounded by railings enclosing a communal garden. The doors of the villas were open from the start, and the garden gates were opened two weeks after the inauguration of the scheme, at the request of the nursing staff. By the time of our survey in 1960 the railings had been removed. The report goes on to describe how mixing between men and women patients was at first permitted to develop spontaneously. In the first week about a dozen male and female patients began associating inside and outside the villas. During the second week a programme of occupational and social activity was introduced, and these arrangements still held in much the same form at the time of our visit in 1960. The patients were divided into groups each under the charge of a particular nurse. The weekly programme included physical training in the main hospital, light gardening, ward cleaning, a drawing and painting class and outdoor games. All activities were conducted on a mixed basis. The organisers had noted the apparent improvement in behaviour of deteriorated patients when they were mixed in social gatherings. In addition there was a social evening with dancing and games once a week and there was also an opportunity to join in dances and cinema shows at the main hospital.

By 1960 the two villas cared for seventy men and women—almost all long-stay schizophrenic patients. The ward restrictiveness score of the villa was low; only 20 per cent.

The patients were much younger than those on Kerry Ward, with an average age of 39 years (none was over 50). Fewer patients had been in hospital for twenty years or more (15 per cent) but the median length of stay was almost the same as on Kerry Ward—thirteen years.

The villas were a few yards apart and a hundred yards or so from the main hospital and surrounded by trees and open space. There was no fence to the hospital and patients could easily walk into the surrounding community. Dormitories were on the upper floors. The three downstairs rooms of Longfield Villa were used as a dining centre, patients sitting at tables for four. The ground floor of the other villa was made up of a large sitting-room, a television room and one other room used for meetings, music groups and indoor games. Most patients had contacts with relatives. Two-thirds were visited in the six months before the survey, and nearly half had gone home on leave during this time.

As on Kerry Ward, six staff were usually on duty from 7.30 a.m. to 8 p.m., working in two shifts. Again, most of the nurses had been on the villas only a relatively short period of time, but they were used quite differently. The introductory leaflet recognised the importance of getting to know patients as quickly as possible and made the following suggestions:

1. 'Distribution of medicine helps you to make contact with the patients and to get to know their names.'

2. One nurse should be responsible for one dining-room, thus supervising only one-third of the total meals.

3. 'Small group meetings (where the nurse with another staff member meets 6 to 8 patients once a week) help you to get to know how patients in such a small group feel and behave.'

4. Each nurse should be associated with an occupational therapy group 'consisting of 12 patients, with whom he or she will work'.

5. Study the ward bed roll, and so become 'familiar with bed positions for each patient'.

Probably the most effective innovation had been the splitting up of the patients into smaller groups with which particular nurses were always associated, accompanying them to occupational therapy and other activities.

The doors of the villas opened directly on to the garden and this gave a sense of freedom in comparison to the main hospital wards. During the lunch period and at other times patients could be seen moving between the two villas and walking about the gardens. From about 7 a.m. to 8.30 p.m. the doors were unlocked and there was little obvious physical control over movement. The bathroom, however, was kept locked and patients were discouraged from going to bed early, especially when evening entertainment was provided, although some discretion was allowed. The sister said that patients often went early when 'mentally relapsed on the day'. One of the twelve patients in our series went to bed at four o'clock on the survey day. All were free to visit the hospital and move about the grounds and, in theory at least, to visit the local village. The sister reported that 16 to 18 of the 35 women went, and that the majority did not ask permission first.

There were restrictions however. Bathing was only allowed on certain days and patients had to wait at the meal tables until tablets had been given out ('to make sure no one is missed'), but in comparison with Kerry Ward the amount of discretion allowed patient and nurse was remarkable. The nurse was not present as a matter of course during bathing: she ran the bath and in most cases then left the patient, but always took the key controlling the bath taps. Six patients washed their own hair and most were allowed to use the kitchen for minor tasks. The sister thought about twenty patients had done something in the kitchen at some time (four of the twelve did so on the day of the survey). 'We don't let them use it *ad lib*. If they don't like the food they may scramble an egg. It has to be well controlled—some of the lost patients can be dangerous.' Patients were allowed to smoke outside the dormitory although the sister said they were told to ask at the meal table whether the others minded them smoking at this time. Many possessed their own matches. Patients were allowed to control the television, and the six patients who showed the most initiative were always there first.

There had been an obvious effort to encourage skills and to allow the nurse initiative in the amount of supervision she exercised. Our research methods were too crude to allow a fully satisfactory evaluation of the policy, but it had clearly had some success. For example, only two of the twelve patients studied intensively needed much by way of help with their toilet. It is easier, however, to evaluate what had been achieved in the matter of personal possessions. Patients were very much better off than in Kerry Ward. Each of the twelve had at least one dress—some had several dresses: all but one had an overcoat, all but three a comb and a toothbrush, all but four some kind of cosmetic and handbag. Only four, however, possessed scissors or a nail file or a mirror. There had been a largely successful effort to return clothing to patients after cleaning. Although not all had personal underclothing, six of the twelve did own some kind of foundation garment. There was plenty of storage space with access at any time but only eighteen wardrobes were provided. Although it was clear that much remained to be done, the women on the whole looked different from those at Severalls. Use of make-up was fairly common, hair was longer and often styled, and the dresses were brighter and better fitting. It seemed to us that the appearance of the majority would not have brought adverse comment in the world outside.

Privacy was, of course, restricted, but the lavatories could be locked, the baths were screened and even the most disturbed patients could (and did) go off alone about the grounds and hospital.

Personal possessions were not commonly to be seen about the ward, although a few things were to be observed. However, the villa was brightly and pleasantly furnished; there were curtains and flowers. Facilities were much better than in Kerry Ward. Each patient had a personal locker, the kitchen could be used, clothes could be washed (although the sister thought the sinks were not big enough), there were two electric irons and two ironing boards, clothes could be sent for dry-cleaning and there were mirrors in each dormitory. Four daily newspapers were provided and seemed to be really available to patients.

There was a definite daily routine, although it was not, as in Kerry Ward, geared mainly to the physical needs of the patients and the ward. The nurses were encouraged to see their job in much broader terms.

Since there was a good deal of variation within the basic time-table, it is easier to convey an idea of a typical day by concentrating on the activities of the twelve women in the series who were studied in detail. Most were up an hour before the day staff came on duty at 7.30 a.m. and had washed and made their beds by 7 a.m. Two of the twelve did not get up until the day staff arrived—one had to be 'pushed into washing' and the other helped by a nurse. Before breakfast at 8.30 a.m. three had got cups of tea from the kitchen and four had done small chores about the villa. Although a few spent their time chatting, we calculated almost half the time before breakfast was spent doing nothing. All had their own tables, and the meal lasted about half an hour. Patients did not leave the table until tablets had been given out.

The week before the survey, separate milk and sugar had been introduced at each table. The sister said that at first most patients had no idea of how to use a teaspoon and that the majority had objected to the change as being too much trouble. In one of the three dining-rooms the nurses were still teaching patients how to use a knife and fork. Food was served at the tables by the nurse helped by one or two patients. Patients were encouraged, before they left, to stack the china on the tables ready for collection.

After breakfast the majority of the women went over to the adjoining villa. Those working on the land (three) went off to a hut in the grounds directly after breakfast, often doing odd jobs about the hut (such as feeding the pet donkey) before starting work. Most went off at ten o'clock to the main occupational therapy building. Before this five did some ward chore (such as washing-up) and a few went off as a group to do a half hour's physical training in the main hospital building. One met her man friend and another wandered about the hospital doing nothing. In all group activities, patients were accompanied by their own nurses who were expected to join in and encourage the patients. The hospital had many different kinds of 'occupational therapy' ranging from typing and high grade industrial work to traditional occupational therapy handicraft. The largest workshop contained both men and women and carried out a variety of jobs brought into the hospital from outside industry: varying from the most simple (dismantling old G.P.O. equipment) to quite complex assembling tasks. Such work had been first introduced in 1957 and everyone seemed agreed that it had produced a better atmosphere—that patients 'had been bored with that arty crafty stuff'. In 1960 several hundred patients were engaged in such work. Nurses stayed throughout the two-hour morning and afternoon sessions to encourage and help their own groups of Longfield patients.

The midday meal lasted half an hour and there was then a one-and-a-half-hour break before work began again at two o'clock. During this time most of the women sat about doing nothing; and they were again largely inactive in the free hour before tea at five o'clock. However, after tea most went along to the 'Health and Beauty class' in the main hospital and joined in the activities (for $1\frac{1}{2}$ hours). One went to the local village with her man friend, one went to bed early and one did nothing (at the P.T. class). There was a brief supper and all twelve were in bed by eight o'clock. The sister said a few on the ward stayed up until ten o'clock watching television, but most were very pleased to go to bed, and went without help.

Different activities were provided on most evenings of the week, including one small discussion group with members of the staff. On Saturday a walk and games were organised, and on Sunday a walk and a visit to the hospital church.

On this ward only one of the twelve selected patients spent most of her time doing 'nothing'. All spent many hours off the ward and in 'useful' activity. The average amount of time spent in inactivity was, of course, relatively low ($4\frac{1}{4}$ hours compared with $7\frac{1}{4}$ hours in Kerry Ward) but relatively few did anything with their 'free time', when not participating in some kind of supervised activity. This must be balanced by the fact that the patients did much more for themselves. Almost all, for example, made their own bed and looked after their own toilet and personal appearance.

The staff were more optimistic about the patients than at Severalls.

For example, the sister thought that nine of the twelve patients could be quite free to visit the local shops when they liked; that eight were able to do useful work for the hospital, that all could possess matches and scissors and half could be allowed to go out with a male patient. The nurses agreed closely on most things. However, the sister thought that a useful female worker in a place like the laundry should receive 7s. 6d. a week (the highest amount received by any of the twelve), while the nurse thought 30s. would be more appropriate, saying that the patients could use the money to buy more clothes and so on. The sister mentioned that some of the patients would benefit from owning more make-up, toothbrushes and toothpaste, handbags and clothing, and when asked what additional facilities she wanted on the ward, mentioned articles of direct concern to the patients—that all should have their own wardrobes, handbags, dressing gowns and slippers. It was difficult in our brief visit to do more than record obvious aspects of ward life, but we thought that such answers reflected a general concern with the needs of the patients as individuals—something not surprising given the avowed aims of the Unit but nonetheless quite different from the answers in Kerry Ward, which were concerned solely with improving the housekeeping equipment. Nurses in Longfield Villa were told that their job was to be with patients and to help them regain earlier skills by encouragement and example. These standards were reinforced in regular discussions at which medical and senior nursing staff were often present. Nurses did work closely with patients during group activities, giving a good deal of personal assistance to those who needed it. One aim, which was fulfilled from time to time, was to bring patients up to the level at which they could be transferred to the Resettlement Villa. A full evaluation of the effectiveness of the programme would have needed a longer and more intensive period of observation. We have noted, however, that the women tended to do nothing when left alone. Nurses were certainly less in evidence during the 'free periods'. This might be considered a shortcoming of the programme; but there had also been an effort on the part of the organisers to resist too great an obtrusiveness into the lives of the patients. To quote the nurses' instructions: 'do not be unduly persuasive where a patient will not enter into these activities (i.e. Physical Training) but rather assist with those who make some sign of joining in'. The staff deliberately intruded a good deal into the patients' day and there was clearly some reluctance to interfere too much with their 'free time', as well as a need on the part of the nurses to withdraw a little at times from the face-to-face contact. The nurses, of course, also took time off themselves for meals and relaxation during these 'free periods'.

The nurses conveyed their belief in the significance of their work and felt it was having some effect. There was also a recognition that more could be done. The sister told us, for example, that she would like to see more action—a greater effort to put more of the things discussed at meetings into effect. The nurses were not uncritical and were very willing to make adverse as well as favourable comments; but, on the whole, morale was high.

During the four years between our visits in 1960 and 1964 there were further important changes. Another ward was added to the complex, and men and women slept in the same villa. The new villa was kept for those needing less supervision, although the same overall programme applied to all three.

The ward restrictiveness score had increased slightly at Longfield in 1964—34 per cent in comparison with the earlier 20 per cent. One patient had been discharged. (She had shown marked poverty of speech and affect in 1960 and had expressed a wish to stay in hospital. However, according to the case-records she had improved considerably.) One, moderately handicapped, patient had been transferred to another hospital. Two other patients were away on holiday at a mental hospital in Devon (they were interviewed on their return). Two patients had been transferred to an intermediate villa at a rather higher level than Longfield and two more were in the Resettlement Unit (one of them was actually working outside hospital). Two patients were on ordinary wards in the main hospital and four were still in the Resocialisation Unit. Eight of the ten patients who were interviewed again in 1964 had improved in clinical condition to some extent during the interim, but one mute patient and one completely incoherent patient had made no progress.

Time spent doing nothing had dropped dramatically from an average of 4 hours 12 minutes per day to just over 2 hours. Of particular note was the increase in leisure activity not organised by the hospital. In 1964 there was a great deal more talking, smoking, reading, writing, walking with men friends, and the like. If organised activities such as physical training are excluded, an average of 21 minutes was spent on 'leisure activity' in 1960 and 2 hours 44 minutes in 1964 (1 hour 46 minutes if visits to the hospital cinema are excluded). The number of personal possessions had more than doubled and the nurses were more positive in their opinions of what the women were able to do—10 positive opinions (out of a possible score of 13) in comparison with 8·7 in 1960. Nine of the ten patients, for example, were thought able to go out with a male patient in 1964, compared with only four in 1960.

SIX PATIENTS IN LONGFIELD VILLA

Longfield patient No. 56. Mrs Olive G

Mrs G was first admitted to hospital in 1938 at the age of 29. She was incoherent in speech, laughed and cried alternately, and said that she was related to royalty. It was impossible to follow her conversation.

At interview in 1960 the main symptom was speech disorder. Asked if her physical health was all right, she replied: 'Doing a lot then still being a right being. It is religion. Good religion. Being religious being as well. I don't know.' She had delusions of various kinds which were difficult to follow because of her incoherence. Her affect was markedly flat (clinical group 3). She had little knowledge of events outside the hospital and did not want to leave. Her appearance was neat and tidy and her hair attractive.

There was considerable improvement by 1964, when Mrs G was able to converse fairly coherently and had only a few fragmentary delusions (clinical group 1*b*). She was well informed about current affairs but had no desire to leave hospital. She had left Longfield Villa and was living in one of the main hospital wards.

Longfield patient No. 65. Miss Sylvia H

Miss H was admitted to hospital in 1944 at the age of 22. She thought she was being persecuted by fifth columnists, and a clinical note in 1952 described her as an 'inaccessible disintegrated schizophrenic'. She remained autistic but denied auditory hallucinations.

At interview in 1960, she was frozen-faced though she once

managed the semblance of a smile, had disordered very short-cut hair and far too much make-up. Her replies were mostly monosyllabic but she became incoherent if she answered at greater length. 'My head gets in the way a little. There's a great deal too much sound. Only in this ward. I'm not sure I've kept up with my head. As soon as I entered I didn't consider my head. There has been a lot of talk. It interrupts the mind' (clinical group 3). She wanted to stay in hospital.

When seen again in 1964 Miss H was very much better. She had moved to the Resettlement Unit and was working in a sheltered factory outside—putting electric elements into blankets. Her conversation was fluent and rational. She discussed the problems of leaving hospital completely realistically and was cautiously in favour of discharge. Her appearance was attractive and, apart from a moderate degree of flattening of affect which still remained, she was very well (clinical group 1*b*).

Longfield patient No. 66. Miss Margery I

Miss I was admitted in 1957 at the age of 20, mute, manneristic and grimacing. Subsequent notes in the case-record described a slow, apathetic girl with little conversation and no initiative, who needed almost everything done for her.

At interview in 1960 she seemed a quiet, scared little thing, with mouth open, eyes moving restlessly about but otherwise sitting absolutely still in her chair. There were long pauses before she answered questions (if at all) and then one or two words would be uttered in a very low voice (clinical group 4). However, she knew the price of a postage stamp and said that she had gone home for Christmas. She did not want to leave hospital. Her personal appearance was pleasant.

She made gradual improvement and was finally able to be discharged home though she did not obtain work.

Longfield patient No. 70. Miss Lola J

Miss J was admitted to hospital in 1945 at the age of 17. She had been agitated and odd in behaviour at home and said she was being persecuted. In hospital, she had behaved as though auditorily hallucinated, was over-active and over-talkative at times, and tended to be very solitary.

At interview in 1960 she talked a good deal, but coherently and to the point. She knew she had been ill and that there were problems in finding somewhere to live outside (her mother was looking for another flat). Her general knowledge was very good, and her appearance smart and attractive. She had no symptoms of schizophrenia (clinical group 1 *a*).

In 1964 she had moved to the Resettlement Unit and was working in the hospital workshop, doing soldering. 'It's not so bad here. It's quite nice. I'm looking foward to the time when I can do a job outside so as I can live at home, be company for my mother. But she's over 70 and very strong-willed.' Miss J had actually worked outside hospital for three months during the previous year but had found the very long journey to and from work too much for her. Her conversation was again very copious, a bit scattered in content, and she seemed slightly puzzled all the time, but on the whole her own judgement of herself was correct. 'There's nothing much wrong with me now. It's just to fit myself in the outside world. I've been in the institution with a crowd of people; I am not so used to mixing outside. I am nervous of travelling outside but I expect I shall manage it all right' (clinical group 1 *a*).

Longfield patient No. 72. Miss Ethel K

Miss K was admitted to hospital from 1940 to 1943 and again in 1947, when she was 21 years old. At the time of the second admission she was mute, muttering unintelligibly to herself, and impulsively aggressive. She had remained mute, inaccessible and incontinent since.

At interview in 1960 she refused to enter the interview room, but her behaviour was observed in other situations. She did not speak at all, but there were frequent lip movements (clinical group 5). She stayed by herself but was able to eat without much supervision and was not incontinent if she was raised at night. Her hair was cut short but otherwise her appearance was reasonable.

In 1964 she presented exactly the same picture. She mumbled occasionally but rarely spoke, and then repeated one word over and over again (clinical group 5). She did very little either in the ward or the occupational therapy department but would occasionally push a polisher aimlessly over the floor, regardless of who was standing in the way. She had to be reminded to wash and use the lavatory.

Longfield patient No. 74. Miss Mary L

Miss L was admitted to hospital in 1940 at the age of 20. She was catatonic, mute, dishevelled in appearance and very slow to move. She sat in one corner all day. After a leucotomy she became over-active, noisy and destructive, with unintelligible speech. In 1957 she was recorded as having visual hallucinations. From 1959, when Stemetil was first begun, she had been more controlled and less withdrawn.

At interview in 1960 she presented an abstracted appearance, leaning forward in her chair but not taking much interest in the conversation. She had a heavy moustache but pleasantly styled hair and a well-fitting dress. Conversation was limited to a few words and she wanted to stay in hospital (clinical group 4). She was fairly well acquainted with current affairs.

In 1964, Miss L was living in a villa intermediate between the Resocialisation and Resettlement Units. She spoke very much more spontaneously about her relatives and prospects of finding work and showed some interest in leaving hospital. She had made measurable progress (clinical group 1*b*).

Downswood Villa

Downswood Villa had been set up in 1957 about the same time as Longfield Villa, with the specific purpose of helping long-stay patients to live and work outside hospital. Many of the long-stay patients who left hospital after 1957 passed through the Unit. It was a large villa in the grounds of the main hospital, with accommodation for 94 patients; these were of both sexes although there was usually a slightly higher proportion of women. Patients were drawn from all parts of the hospital and were on the whole much less disturbed than those on the two wards so far described. Before they were considered for the Unit they had to have been in the hospital at least two years, 'to be relatively stabilised and socially acceptable, have reasonable current work records in the hospital and be under the age of 55'. The aims of the Unit have always been clear: 'to review the capacity of the patients for work and social adjustment, and to encourage as many of them as possible to live partially or wholly in the community outside hospital, with or without some sheltered accommodation or employment'. By 1960 the work of the Unit was well established.

Under the influence of workers such as Maxwell Jones some attempt had been made from the start to modify the status differences between staff and between staff and patients within the hospital; 'to delegate more responsibility, and encourage the expression of individual views and the practice of making joint decisions'. Each day the nurses worked in two 'shifts'. At the time of the survey a male charge nurse and a female student nurse took one and a sister and a male staff nurse took the other. A consultant psychiatrist who worked part-time on the Unit was leader of the team and there was a full-time psychiatric social worker. There were two regular weekly meetings for the staff. An assistant matron and an assistant chief male nurse kept contact with the nursing side, and a male and female occupational therapist formed a link with the patients' work situation in the hospital. A disablement resettlement officer from the local employment exchange attended one of the weekly meetings, which was mainly devoted to the assessment of patients considered for work outside the hospital. On admission to the Unit an up-to-date social history was completed and, in the light of other information provided by the staff, possibilities for the employment and resettlement of each patient were discussed. The outlook for patients entering the Unit was reasonably good. In the first three to four years 210 patients had been admitted to the Unit: of these 21 per cent had been discharged and not re-admitted, and 23 per cent were working outside the hospital but living in the Unit.

There were also meetings for patients and staff. A general ward meeting was held fortnightly which was attended by staff on duty and patients; ward problems were discussed and films shown. At the time of the survey not all patients attended and it had been decided that this should not be made obligatory unless by the patients' own decision as a group.

The patients were also divided into six groups of fifteen for the purpose of meetings held regularly for an hour each week. Two staff members were allocated to each group. Topics discussed largely covered matters to do with everyday living within the hospital and the ward, and problems of leaving the hospital and earning a living. The discussion of personal problems was rare. Various other activities were organised (there was a party the week of the survey) but there were a good deal fewer of these than in Longfield Villa.

Almost all the forty-eight women living in the Villa at the time of the survey had been diagnosed as schizophrenic. Their average age was 41 (the eldest was 56) and their average length of stay was eight years. Only one patient had been in hospital as long as twenty years, but one-third had been in at least ten years.

There was a ten-minute walk down a steep hill to get to the local village, shops and buses for nearby towns. The Villa had an attractive garden and was surrounded by shrubs and trees. The main buildings could not be easily seen and there was nothing that was obviously 'institutional' about the building or its setting. The ground floor contained the main living area; and might well have been part of a reasonably good hotel.

The ward restrictiveness score was low—14 per cent. The doors were opened very early (some of the patients working outside hospital left before 7 a.m.) and were not locked by the night staff until nearly 11 p.m. Movement about the building was largely unrestricted and the men and women sat together in the day-rooms. The kitchen was locked at eight o'clock when the day staff went off duty, and the female half of the villa was locked during the night. There was a sense of freedom about the place that was clearly genuine—patients came and went as they pleased. All went about the hospital and grounds alone and most visited the local village (all without needing to ask permission). But there were quite explicit rules and restrictions. Most of these were a considered part of the organisation of the Unit: it was felt that patients must develop responsible and regular habits that would fit them for life outside. Times of morning rising and meal attendance were clearly laid down: drugs were given out in the sister's office only at certain times and it was insisted that ward chores and washing-up rotas were strictly adhered to. Patients were expected to be punctual in attending their various places of work. Lying in bed during the day was strictly forbidden. By the time of our second visit in 1964 these rules had been printed on posters and displayed in the Unit. A roll call was taken at 8 p.m., when all were required to be in the Unit unless in possession of a late pass authorised by the doctor; after this they could go out about the hospital (to get cigarettes from the slot-machine, for example) but not out of the grounds. The night nurse called about 10.30 p.m., gave out sedatives and locked up for the night.

All these rules had been discussed with the patients at the various Unit meetings and were an accepted part of life in the Villa. There were other restrictions, however, which were apparently vestiges of the past. For example, the bathroom was left open after tea until eight o'clock, on Wednesday afternoons and most of Saturday and Sunday. But a bath-key had to be used to turn the taps and this had to be collected from the sister's office. (One of our patients came into the crowded office while we were there to ask the charge nurse for it.) Once collected, the key remained freely available until the bathroom was shut at night. The doors of the bathroom could be locked. The rule about the bath-tap key appeared to be left over from the old hospital regulations, but the nurse we spoke to about it saw no reason for giving it up. Two of the baths were in the same room and were not screened; this had been brought up at meetings and complained about 'umpteen times' to the hospital authorities but nothing had been done. Smoking was not allowed at meal-times—'we get complaints: they use saucers as ash trays. We do not allow smoking in the dining-room.' When the Villa had been taken over, some of the former staff and patients remained and it would, perhaps, have been remarkable if the influence of the main institution had not been seen in many ways. Nonetheless the amount of responsibility allowed to patients was considerable. They were responsible for regulating their day and particularly for getting to meals and work on time, collecting their medicine, for their own toilet and bed-making, seeing to their own laundry and repairing their clothes. All had small chores such as washing-up to do. They were allowed to use the kitchen for small things such as boiling an egg or making tea. Although attendance at meetings was voluntary there was a general expectation that patients should go.

Life on the ward was more varied than in Longfield, and the most satisfactory way of conveying something of this is to deal with the sixteen women studied intensively. All but two were up when the day-staff came on duty at 7.30 a.m. Two were up at six o'clock, got their own breakfast and had left by seven o'clock to work in a nearby town. Three others were just about to start an eight-week course at a government Industrial Rehabilitation Unit some fifteen miles from the hospital. All looked after their own toilet and made their beds without help. Of the fourteen who remained in the hospital, one got her own breakfast ('she is fussy about the hospital food'), while the rest collected food between 8.00 and 8.15 and took no longer than fifteen minutes over eating it. About half collected tablets from the sister's office afterwards: sometimes they had to wait a few minutes in a small queue. All did some ward chore lasting 30 to 45 minutes before they went off to work. Six did domestic work about the hospital (mainly on other wards): three were in the main hospital kitchen: two did industrial work, two typing and clerical work, and one worked in the hospital sewing room. Most worked about five hours (but a few for considerably longer—one for nine hours) and had a midday break of two hours. No more than half an hour was spent at lunch. For these patients it was more difficult to judge time spent unoccupied. Two were said, for example, to listen to the wireless. However, the most cautious estimate suggested that few were unoccupied, in marked contrast to Longfield in 1960. Most read or knitted, but only two were said to do much talking; two went straight back to work and only four of the fourteen sat about doing nothing. After tea, which was at five o'clock, patients were left to their own devices. The most common activity was watching television (about a third of the time) but a good deal of time was spent on personal chores such as washing clothes; reading, walking and knitting were also quite common. Again, relatively little time was spent unoccupied: for the whole day it was an average of one and a half hours (four and a quarter in Longfield and seven and a quarter on Kerry). Only three of the sixteen patients spent as long as three hours completely unoccupied. All were off the ward for a good deal of the day. Three went for long walks in the grounds or to the local village, two of these with men friends; but the amount of mixing and talking with others was almost certainly small. When we visited the Villa most patients were to be seen watching television or engaged in some more or less solitary pursuit. By usual standards they went to bed early, half by nine o'clock and only a quarter later than 10.30 p.m.

Personal possessions were much more common than on the other two wards. Each had at least one dress (usually several), an overcoat, a comb, a toothbrush, handbag and some personal ornament. All had at least three sets of underwear and some kind of foundation garment.

All but one had make-up, all but two had a mirror and all but three scissors or a nail file. At least in the range and quantity of their possessions little seemed to be wanting. It was a part of the Unit's policy for patients to work for a time from the hospital before an attempt was made to resettle them fully. This, to quote a hospital report, 'gives them an opportunity to establish themselves firmly in employment, to make good their deficiencies in clothes and belongings, and to allow relatives and the Unit staff to gain more confidence in their rehabilitation'.

Facilities on the whole were good. There was ample opportunity for washing clothes—basins, airing rails, electric iron, etc. Only a few had hospital clothes (which were used for work) and all were expected to wash their own. They could get clothes dry-cleaned outside the hospital by filling in a form. There were fifty-one lockers for the women but only three wardrobes. The latter seemed the main short-coming—there were fourteen feet of curtained railing in one of the corridors. There was a very well-stocked lending library in a nearby villa and also a hairdresser—patients were allowed one free shampoo and set a month.

The nurses were optimistic and in close agreement about what they thought the patients could do—the sister scored an average of 12·1 out of a possible 13 on the opinion statements. Ten of the sixteen were thought able to work outside hospital while living in the Unit, and seven able to leave if suitable accommodation could be found.

Neither of the two nurses thought that the hospital supplied all the patients' requirements—party clothes, cinema, make-up, soap, stationery, hairdresser, books, magazines and outings were things they were felt to need money for. However, the women received only an average of 7s. 6d. a week from the hospital. When asked, the sister thought a worker should receive 20s. a week, while the nurse thought 7s. 6d.; but when specifically asked about each patient in turn they mentioned, on average, much the same amount as each other—about 10s. Asked what additional facilities she would like, the sister mentioned 'a bit more modern kitchen, a ward orderly, seven modern mops and brooms, and more modern furniture'—she thought what they had was drab. She did not think they had much difficulty in keeping order. 'I find just talking is usually enough. I explain that they made the rules [at meetings] and it's up to them to keep them. I've stopped breakfast once or twice when someone has been late. They are much better than I ever thought they would be, as chronic as they are.' Like others we spoke to on the ward, she had no doubts about what she was doing—'rehabilitation—make them socially acceptable outside; and make life more worth while inside if they can't manage it outside...it [the Unit] has done good'.

Four years later, six of the sixteen had been discharged (one of them married a male patient from the Villa) and two were working outside hospital but living in. A further four had shown some improvement in mental state and one some deterioration. Seven were still in a Rehabilitation Unit (another had been opened): there had been no change in their social withdrawal scores (which were already low) but the amount of time spent doing nothing had dropped from 1 hour 49 minutes to 1 hour 4 minutes. Scanning of time budgets does not suggest any dramatic changes in their lives. One had a man friend where none was mentioned before. There was, however, a marked tendency to get to bed earlier—at nine o'clock on average instead of 10.15.

SIX DOWNSWOOD PATIENTS

Downswood patient No. 17. Miss Elizabeth M

Miss M was first admitted in 1953 when she was aged 28. At that time she thought her mother was trying to poison her. She was re-admitted in 1956 complaining of telepathic communications. She said she was married and wore a ring. She showed odd mannerisms.

At interview in 1960 she spoke well and rationally but tended to return to one topic only—that of her real name and whether she was married or not. She hoped she would leave hospital eventually 'to return to my husband' who would have 'to sue for my release through the law courts' (she was not under any legal restriction). Her personal appearance was good but there was moderate blunting of affect (clinical group 2).

In 1964, Miss M was living in the Resettlement Villa. Her affect and speech were normal and she simply said that she didn't know whether she was married or not. Of her previous symptoms she said, 'It is like a dream when you are awake' (clinical group 1*a*). Her appearance was smart, and she had applied make-up skilfully. She said she was reasonably content in hospital but would be prepared to leave if she found a good enough job. She was doing clerical work but was slow at it. Her father was over 80 and she hated the idea of digs: a hostel would be better.

Downswood patient No. 18. Mrs Georgia N

Mrs N was admitted for a few months during 1949, when she had a leucotomy, and then again in 1950 when she was aged 39. It was said that she had a 'persecution complex', heard remarks in 'the other seven languages' and had been ill at least since 1943. She thought that details of her personal life were broadcast on the radio. She was divorced in 1956.

In 1960 her conversation was quite incoherent. 'As regards finance how would I gain any benefit over this thing called espionage? I think over some months I should receive some hundreds in small amounts. But the numbers are important.' Her affect was markedly flat (clinical group 3). However her hair, make-up and personal appearance were attractive. Her attitude to discharge could not be rated because of incoherent speech.

In 1964 the situation was similar. Asked whether she was content to stay in hospital, Mrs N replied, 'Not a case of content. Might be possible. You would have a certainty of citizenship in accordance with marriage licence from which point we might negotiate...' 'Some people will leave in due course when the churches are exempted. Others are here to oppose me. They are doing their best to cheat the crown' (clinical group 3). Her appearance was still smart and attractive.

Downswood patient No. 26. Miss Joyce O

Miss O was admitted in 1955 when she was aged 24. She said that the girls at work had been talking about her, she had neglected her personal cleanliness and become solitary.

At interview in 1960 she seemed bored and there was moderate flattening of affect and poverty of speech. Otherwise there were no symptoms (clinical group 1b). Her hair was greasy and unstyled, she had no make-up and her general appearance was dowdy. She said she wanted to leave but had no plans for what she would do. She was in fact discharged home on 13 June 1960.

Downswood patient No. 28. Mrs Dora P

Mrs P was admitted in 1941 at the age of 36 and transferred to her current hospital in 1945. She had been divorced before admission. She said she had led an immoral life, that she frequently met Lawrence of Arabia, that there were ten substitutes for her husband and that she heard voices abusing her. She was leucotomised in 1945. She wrote many strange letters to insurance companies during the early years of her stay.

At interview in 1960, Mrs P was haughty and aloof but otherwise pleasant in manner. She thought that her visitors were all impostors arranged by the hospital and she had a range of other delusions (clinical group 2). She wanted to leave but was unrealistic in her plans to be a dentist's receptionist. Her appearance was neat and smart.

In 1964, she was much more realistic in her assessment of the chances of discharge. She was working outside hospital, packing soap. She was still preoccupied with certain past events (she thought that she had been swindled out of large sums of money) but was less actively preoccupied (clinical group 2). Her appearance was still smart.

Downswood patient No. 31. Miss Dorothy Q

Miss Q had been admitted in 1952 at the age of 40. She was then 'domineering, cantankerous and argumentative'. She complained vaguely of various somatic influences and lived on bread and tea in order to control them. She was untidy and withdrawn and thought that everyone in the neighbourhood was against her.

At interview in 1960 she was very suspicious and evaded answering many questions: 'I must answer that with reserve.' She thought that psychiatrists had been responsible for her previous bodily symptoms and they were now trying to undo the harm they had done (clinical group 2). She was fairly resigned to staying in hospital but did not want to say so without qualification—'It's a very difficult question. I can't answer it.' She visited home regularly and her appearance was attractive.

In 1964 she was no longer in the Rehabilitation Villa. She still made many complaints and was extremely suspicious about every question asked. There was pressure of talk with very little content.

However, she did not actually mention any delusions (clinical group 1*a*). Her personal appearance was less smart but her white hair was well brushed. She said she wanted to leave, but put forward many reasons why she did not.

Downswood patient No. 33. Miss Laura R

Miss R was admitted to hospital in 1948 for insulin coma and then again in 1954 when she was 45. She said she had a spiritual attachment to an organist who could put thoughts into the minds of others. She heard voices and thought people stared at her. Since that time she had been vague, flat and indecisive, but occasionally became depressed and wept.

At interview in 1960 she was tearful and depressed. She said she was getting farther away from God. People sometimes seemed to say the same thing as she was thinking and their voices did not appear to belong to them. From time to time she was aurally hallucinated (clinical group 2). She wanted to stay in hospital. Her general appearance was good.

In 1964 she was still perplexed and vague and probably deluded and hallucinated. ('Anything like hypnotism going on?' 'Such things are possible. I have noticed certain things', but she was unable to elaborate.) She had not heard voices recently. Her affect was moderately flat and there was moderate poverty of speech (clinical group 2). Her general appearance was excellent. She had a vague wish to leave hospital: 'It's very difficult to say. Times when you'd like to and others when you wouldn't.' She was no longer living in the Rehabilitation Villa.

Discussion

We undertook more detailed study of the living conditions of all the wards containing 20 per cent or more of patients in the series and some of this material has been presented in an earlier chapter as 'ward restrictiveness' scores. Inevitably, we retained general impressions of the wards, the staff and the patients which were not quantifiable but provided us with some understanding of how the hospitals were functioning. Other observers spending time in these three hospitals, even if they were making the same systematic observations, might well have come away with different conclusions. It is very easy to be unfair to hardworking and dedicated staff, themselves working under conditions of neglect and lack of interest from the world outside, and it is also easy to underestimate the extent to which apparently apathetic patients are aware of social deprivations because they do not complain.

We considered whether to present this extra descriptive material at some length but decided, partly because the book would become twice as long but largely on scientific grounds, that it would be best to derive our conclusions mainly from the data that could be quantified, drawing upon our impressions only for the more speculative sections of the final chapter. The three wards described here are probably sufficient illustration of the range of social conditions in the hospitals and we would ask our readers to exercise their imagination in order to give body to the figures which systematically describe the rest of the patients in the series and the social conditions in which they were living.

We shall try, in the final chapter, to bring the conclusions together and to offer some simple interpretations.

9

COMPARATIVE SURVEY
OF SCHIZOPHRENIC PATIENTS IN AN
AMERICAN COUNTY HOSPITAL, 1964

In February 1964 one of the authors was invited by Professor Martin Loeb to spend a few days in Madison, Wisconsin, as a consultant to the County Mental Hospital Project.

The Wisconsin public hospital services differ from those available in other states in the U.S.A. in that a substantial proportion of patients who need long-term care live in small county institutions rather than large state hospitals. Intensive treatment facilities are not available and patients who require these are transferred back to the state hospital. Thirty-six of the 71 Wisconsin counties are served by such institutions, ranging in size from 40 to 380 beds in 1961. Nearly half the patients had been in hospital for more than ten years.

The hospital chosen for the present study was Columbia County Hospital, Wyocena. There were 110 male and 215 female patients on 1 July 1960, 22 per cent of them classified as mentally subnormal, the rest as mentally ill. Thirty-six per cent of patients had a diagnosis of schizophrenia. Three-quarters had been transferred from a state institution and 19 per cent were direct admissions. Forty per cent had been resident for ten years or more. All patients were committed, as there was no form of voluntary or non-statutory admission.

The superintendent and matron were a married couple with no professional training. The attendants had no qualification in psychiatric nursing but there was a part-time social worker.

The Columbia County Hospital could not strictly be compared with any of the three British hospitals. However, it was thought that the same measurements of clinical and social conditions should be applied at Columbia County, in order to see whether there were any problems about administration in a different cultural setting, and to make a crude comparison with the data available at Mapperley in 1964. This would at least indicate whether more sophisticated comparative work might be possible.

The selection criteria were exactly the same as for the British

[166]

hospital, except that both men and women were interviewed, since numbers were so small. Forty-five patients, 21 men and 24 women, fitted the selection criteria for the study and all but one man, who declined, were seen.

DIAGNOSIS

It was possible to make a definite diagnosis of schizophrenia, on the basis of the clinical interview together with information from the case-notes, in only 11 men and 18 women. There was some evidence of schizophrenia, but not enough for a clear diagnosis, in 4 men. For 2 men and 2 women there was no specific evidence for or against the diagnosis. One woman, who showed no specific symptoms at examination, had had an illness which, as described in the case-record, could have been schizophrenia or mania.

In the remaining 6 patients, 3 men and 3 women, a diagnosis other than schizophrenia could fairly confidently be made, according to the system of diagnosis generally taught in Britain. Two men had had Delirium Tremens and one Depression. The three women had all suffered from forms of Depression. These 6 patients have been excluded from the subsequent analysis. The remaining patients have been included, although several of them may not be suffering from schizophrenia according to the criteria used for the British surveys.

AGE AND LENGTH OF STAY

Age was much the same in the two series—just over half the patients in each group were aged 51 to 60. The length of stay of the American patients (including the period at a state mental hospital which normally preceded transfer), although similar for men and women, was shorter than that of the English patients (see Table 9.1, p. 245).

Since the distribution of a length of stay is, in general, much the same in American and British state mental hospitals, these figures indicate a selective transfer to Columbia County Hospital.

UNMATCHED COMPARISONS

(a) *Clinical classification*

Table 9.2 (p. 246) shows that the differences in mental state, crudely classified at the time of examination, are not great.

(*b*) *Ward behaviour scores*

The mean S.W. and S.E. scores are shown in the table below. There were no significant differences.

			S.W.	S.E.
Columbia County:	Men	(N 17)	4·00	1·11
	Women	(N 21)	3·67	1·33
	Total	(N 38)	3·82	1·23
Mapperley	Women	(N 66)	3·09	1·29

(*c*) *Attitude to discharge*

The results are shown in Table 9.3 (p. 246). The distributions were almost identical.

(*d*) *General knowledge*

Fifty-nine per cent of the American patients and 36 per cent of the British patients gave the name of President or Prime Minister correctly. The difference is significant at the 5 per cent level.

About a third of each group gave both the month and the year correctly.

(*e*) *Height and weight*

Apart from the greater height of the American women (which is consistent with population trends in this age-range) there is no significant difference between the series. A small group of ten British women who are 63" or less in height but weigh 191 lbs, or more, has no counterpart in the American series.

(*f*) *Drug administration*

Ten of the men, and 16 of the women at Columbia County Hospital were receiving drug treatment, as were 59 of the 66 women in Mapperley.

The average daily dose, in arbitrary units, taken by those who were receiving drugs is shown in the table below. Thus the British women were receiving rather higher doses (but more drugs were prescribed at Mapperley than at Netherne and Severalls, which were both closer to the Columbia County Hospital practice in this respect).

		Chlor-promazine	Stelazine	Melleril	Nardil
Columbia County:	Men	2·8	2·0	4·5	3·2
	(N)	(6)	(3)	(2)	(3)
	Women	3·0	3·0	1·1	2·1
	(N)	(15)	(2)	(5)	(2)
Mapperley	Women	4·8	5·4	2·3	2·5
	(N)	(39)	(16)	(12)	(2)

Only one patient, at Mapperley, was given E.C.T. during the week before the survey.

(g) *Personal possessions of the patients*

Table 9.4 (p. 247) shows that both series of patients were well equipped with items of clothing (in marked contrast to patients in many other hospitals both in the United States and the United Kingdom). The Americans had more toilet articles such as make-up, scissors, nail file or mirror. The latter instruments are potentially dangerous, but in fact there has been no problem in allowing their use. The American hospital is far more liberal in this respect than the British.

(h) *Attitudes and opinions of nurses or attendants*

Columbia County Hospital had no nurse with a psychiatric training, but attendants were asked the same questions as nurses in the British hospitals. Table 9.5 (p. 247) shows a general similarity in the overall pattern of results, but certain differences stand out. The Columbia County Hospital attendants seem to assume that patients could reach a higher working standard, though the British patients were actually doing slightly more responsible work—see Section (*j*).

Attitudes to money are much as expected. The British patients do in fact receive more money: there is a payment for work done and an allowance of 10*s*. a week for patients who are unable to work. There is, of course, no charge under the National Health Service, whereas the American patients, if discharged, are theoretically supposed to pay their bill. Netherne is a good example of a hospital which has introduced industrial work on a large scale, for which patients are paid at the usual rate for the job.

Mapperley has no locked wards and the nurses' attitudes reflect this. (See also Sections (*i*) and (*l*).)

Very few patients in British mental hospitals are now under any form of legal order. All the American patients were committed and the attendants were not familiar with any other system.

Although many male patients at Columbia County Hospital could theoretically go out with female patients (in practice they were not allowed to do so) the attendants thought that only 24 per cent of women might go out with male patients. In fact there was a system of fairly strict supervision of the female patients, who were not allowed out of the hospital except with relatives or under escort. Most patients at Mapperley, both male and female, could mix with the opposite sex, and many had their regular women-friends or men-friends with whom they would go into town.

(i) *Contact with world outside*

The nurses and attendants provided information about the visitors that patients had received, the visits they had made home and the 'privileges' they were allowed, during the previous six months (Table 9.6, p. 248).

The difference in the frequency that the patients are visited is not striking. The British patients go home rather more often. The main difference, however, lies in the extent to which parole privileges are granted. No patient in the Columbia County Hospital series was allowed town privileges, as against just over one-third at Mapperley. Only 5 per cent of the women had ground privileges, compared with 53 per cent at Mapperley. (It should also be remembered that ground parole at Mapperley was virtually a licence for the patient to go outside the hospital if she wished. No doors are locked, there are no gates and only a low boundary wall.) Ninety-five per cent of women in the County Hospital series were allowed outside the ward only under supervision, compared with 12 per cent at Mapperley.

(j) *Work*

The scores on occupation were as follows:

Columbia County:	Men	5·88
	Women	4·33
	Total	5·03
Mapperley	Women	5·47

These scores indicate that Columbia County women are given rather less responsibility than the men there, or than women at Mapperley. The differences are not great.

(k) Time budget

Table 9.7 (p. 248) shows the difference in time budget.

Apart from details, there are no differences of note in this table. The mean time doing nothing (3·3–4·3 hours per day) is fairly high at both hospitals. (At Netherne it was only 2·8 hours, but at Severalls in 1960 it was 5·7 hours.) In this respect, as in many others, Columbia County and Mapperley come somewhere between an outstandingly good British hospital and another which was average.

The scores on work responsibility (Section *j*) were somewhat higher for women at Mapperley, owing to the presence of a larger proportion of patients who worked outside hospital, in hospital industry or in hospital maintenance departments (laundry, etc.) without supervision. Mapperley also made rather more use of occupational therapy.

(l) Ward restrictiveness

It will be remembered that the range of ward restrictiveness scores was from 0 to 50. The scores at Columbia County Hospital were as follows:

Ward F1	30	M1	29
F2	27	M2	12
F3	25		
F4	18		
F5	19		

Summing these scores according to the numbers of series patients in each ward and dividing by the total number of patients gives an average score of 20·3 (men only, 17·0; women only, 22·9). This figure represents the restrictiveness of ward routine experienced by all the patients in the series, i.e. it takes account of their numerical distribution in the seven wards.

The equivalent average for Mapperley women was 11·9 (ward range from 7 to 15). Thus restrictions were markedly greater in the American than in the British hospital, so far as schizophrenic patients are concerned. Even the men in Columbia County Hospital were more restricted than the British women. These results confirm the differences in parole status described in Section (*i*).

However, the restrictiveness scores do not reach the very high range which is common in some British mental hospital wards (and probably in state mental hospital wards also). At Severalls, in 1964, most of the wards in which the patients in the series were living had scores ranging between 28 and 43.

MATCHED COMPARISONS

Age and length of stay

Since most of the variables under discussion are correlated with length of stay, 38 British patients were selected out of the 66 at Mapperley because they were closest to their American counterparts in this respect. They had still, however, been five years longer in hospital, on average. This procedure also provided matching for age, though the British patients were on average four years older.

The distribution within clinical groups is shown in Table 9.8 (p. 249), which shows that there are rather more patients at Mapperley with no symptoms when length of stay is matched.

The mean S.W. score is 2·3 for the 38 British patients compared with 3·9 for the American, a significant difference. The S.E. scores (1·4 and 1·3) are no different.

Matching for clinical condition

When clinical grouping is matched, instead of length of stay, the mean S.W. scores became equivalent (3·9 in Madison, 3·4 in Nottingham). Mean occupation scores are also equal (5·0 and 5·3) but mean scores representing contact with the outside remain significantly different (3·4 and 6·0).

Discussion

A pattern emerges fairly clearly from these results. Both hospitals provide good material conditions for their patients, who are well clothed, fed and housed. Many of the opinions expressed by nurses and attendants are liberal and tolerant. The patient's day is taken up with constructive activities and leisure pursuits (the American women tend to watch television in the evenings while the British women retire to bed, but this may be a cultural difference!).

There are no standards for comparison with other American hospitals but it seems probable that Columbia County is well above average in all these respects. Certainly, by British standards, Mapperley (and therefore Columbia County) is better than average.

The differences between the two hospitals—particularly in the social conditions experienced by the two groups of women—seem to be due mainly to a different view of public attitudes to mental illness: perhaps these attitudes were even shared by staff. The female American patients are regarded as in the need of protection, whatever their clinical condition. Although the attendants said that several could work outside hospital, none in fact did so, because the others would be jealous, or because it would be administratively inconvenient, or because public opinion would not stand for it. There was no such feeling at Mapperley, where the judgement was based only on whether the nurse thought the patient well enough to work outside (four patients actually were doing so). The same considerations applied to town privileges, which were not granted to any of the Americans, while 35 per cent of the British women were able to go into town by themselves. The opinion of nurses and attendants about whether a woman could be trusted to associate with a male patient showed a similar difference—five of the twenty-one American women were regarded as trustworthy compared with twice that proportion of the British women. The practice was even more divergent. Matching for clinical condition did not remove the differences.

The ward restrictiveness scores (an average of 11·9 for the British women against 22·9 for the American women) sum up the major difference between the two hospitals. None of the wards in Columbia County Hospital, even those which were locked, came into the 'very highly restrictive' range, though probably many in a state mental hospital (and in some British mental hospitals) would do so. The pattern was more of external, rather than internal, restrictiveness, but the routine was considerably more relaxed in Mapperley.

How far this basic divergence is, in fact, dependent on public attitudes, or to the interpretation by the staff of what they thought public attitudes might be, cannot emerge from the data presented here, which are purely internal. It might be suggested, however, that a hospital which is largely run by non-professional staff is less insulated from public attitudes and will show greater deference to them. It is true that, in the past, custodial attitudes were commonplace in British mental hospitals and that they still exist in certain hospitals which have not been affected by the recent wind of change, so that the relationship is not a necessary one. However, given the change of attitude which has taken place among a section of the educated public, which is shared by most professionals in Britain (and a substantial group in the United States), it may be easier to introduce changes, and to withstand criticism, if the hospital is run by professionals.

It may be suggested that the rural setting of Columbia County Hospital, compared with Mapperley which is placed on a main road in an industrial city, means that the influences on the two staffs are different, and that this may explain the divergence of practice. In fact, however, the first hospital in Britain to open all its doors—Dingleton Hospital in Scotland—is situated in a rural area. Dr Bell, the superintendent, had to face considerable local opposition, but he was confident enough, and had status enough, to be able to overcome it. Dr Macmillan independently began the same process at Mapperley in 1932, and opened the last ward in 1952 (well before the new drugs were introduced).

It would be pointless, in view of the probable selection biasses, to discuss the similarities in the clinical condition of the two groups of patients, except to remark that Mapperley patients were expected to show greater morbidity than patients in Columbia County Hospital because of selective admissions but, if anything, turned out to have fewer symptoms. Still less is it worthwhile to consider the clinical results in terms of the social differences.

It may, however, be useful to make one or two further observations on matters which were not the subject of systematic quantification. One major difference between the hospitals particularly calls for comment: Columbia County Hospital has very little contact with other psychiatric agencies or services, whereas Mapperley is the centre of a complex network of community services. The psychiatrists at Mapperley work more in the community than they do in hospital. They staff out-patient clinics, they provide a consultative service to local general hospitals, to the local courts and the local Industrial Rehabilitation Unit, they visit many patients in their homes and they keep close contact with general practitioners. The hospital and local authority social workers undertake very similar duties—they meet regularly at case conferences, they see many patients before admission to hospital, they supervise the community care of patients after they are discharged, and they carry out social work with many patients who never come into hospital. Even the hospital nurses are now beginning to provide a home nursing service which should prove most valuable. The extent to which this range of integrated services, based on the mental hospital, actually reduced psychiatric morbidity, is itself the subject of investigation, but the overall pattern is strikingly different from that in Columbia County.

The difference is the more remarkable in that the County Hospital system in Wisconsin (if Columbia County Hospital is typical) would seem to be ideally suited to provide a comprehensive local service. There are, of course, difficulties in providing adequate out-patient facilities, sufficient psychiatrists and social workers with the requisite training and interest, and close co-ordination with other medical and social services. It would be presumptuous to comment on these problems here.

Summary

Only two conclusions are permissible.

The first is that a full-scale comparative survey of the kind outlined here is feasible. The problems of sampling are not insuperable and it should be possible, for example, to see all the in-patients from one or several counties whichever hospital they are currently in. Comparisons between hospitals should be at least as informative as those made between British mental hospitals, given the same attention to admission and discharge rates, and paying due regard to measurable demographic and social factors, such as age, length of stay, social class, etc. Under these conditions tentative hypothesis testing might be possible even using international comparisons. The range of social conditions (and therefore the range of possible 'natural experiments') would certainly be extended.

The second conclusion is that Columbia County Hospital provides, in many respects, a material environment which is above that of the average British mental hospital, equivalent to that of one particular British hospital which has an international reputation for the excellence of its services, and probably well above that of American state mental hospitals. There are, however, restrictive practices which have less counterpart in a good British hospital, even one which deals with the full range of psychiatric disorders, both acute and chronic, from its local community.

INSTITUTIONALISM AND SCHIZOPHRENIA: SUMMARY, DISCUSSION AND CONCLUSIONS

The various stages of this study point towards a conclusion which is very difficult to resist—that a substantial proportion, though by no means all, of the morbidity shown by long-stay schizophrenic patients in mental hospitals is a product of their environment. The social pressures which act to produce this extra morbidity can to some extent be counteracted, but the process of reform may itself have a natural history and an end. We should like, in this final chapter, to discuss these propositions in detail, both in their theoretical and in their practical aspects, and also to consider their implications for the future of mental hospitals and related services.

We put forward, in Chapter 1, three theories which help to predict how schizophrenic patients will react in various social environments. The first differentiated three types of impairment which contribute to the end-state seen in chronic schizophrenia—'premorbid', 'primary' and 'secondary'. The second was concerned with the ways in which 'primary' impairments might vary under different types of social influence. The third dealt with the origin and modification of 'secondary' impairments. The first part of our discussion will focus on certain hypotheses derived from these theories which we have been able to put to the test.

Interaction between clinical and social factors

POVERTY OF THE SOCIAL ENVIRONMENT AS A CAUSE OF CLINICAL DETERIORATION

The most important hypothesis under test is that certain aspects of the social environment actually cause clinical improvement or deterioration. The first step was to show, in Chapter 4, that, looked at from the patient's point of view, there was a certain uniformity in level of social stimulation. Those who had fewest personal possessions tended to be occupied in the least interesting activities, to be regarded most pessimistically by nurses, to be least in touch with the world outside through letters or visits from relatives or weekends at home, and to spend most time doing absolutely nothing. Conversely, those who were best off according to one index, tended also to be well off according to the others. There was a wide range of social experience in each of the hospitals, but in 1960 Severalls patients were likely to be most deprived. (Even there, however, one ward had previously been set aside for private patients and the atmosphere was still not unlike that of a genteel boarding-house.)

Environmental poverty, measured in these terms, was very highly correlated with a 'clinical poverty syndrome', independently measured, and compounded of social withdrawal, flatness of affect and poverty of speech. Both environmental and clinical poverty became more intense with length of stay, although they remained highly interrelated when length of stay was allowed for.

The second step was to show in Chapter 5 that, although the association between clinical and social poverty remained strong in three different mental hospitals, the one with the richest social environment (Netherne) contained patients with the fewest negative symptoms. Even when twenty patients in each hospital were selected because they were equivalent in clinical grouping, degree of social withdrawal, age, length of stay and attitude to discharge, most of the environmental indices still showed Severalls at a disadvantage.

If the negative symptoms do indeed reflect a fundamental process in schizophrenia and have an important biological component, as was suggested in Chapter 1, it might well be assumed that the direction of cause and effect is from patient to environment; that schizophrenia inevitably creates its own social community. To some extent, this must be so if the staff allow it. Thus, if more severely-ill patients had been admitted to Severalls, they might have given rise to at least part of the difference in social environments. We could not demonstrate that schizophrenic patients admitted to Severalls were any more severely ill than those admitted to Netherne or Mapperley; in fact, the discharge rates of the latter two hospitals were higher, which would work in the opposite direction. Nevertheless, the argument is not conclusive.

Even supposing, however, that the poorer results at Severalls in 1960 were really due to more severely-ill patients being originally admitted there, a test of the social hypothesis is still possible.

If schizophrenic patients are 'vulnerable' to under-stimulating social environments (this being one of their most characteristic impairments), they will react by increased withdrawal even to an environment they have created themselves. An attempt can then be made to reverse the process by appropriate staff action. If the social milieu does improve measurably, there should be a corresponding decrease in 'clinical poverty'. This should be true, not only at Severalls, but at the other hospitals as well.

We had every reason to suppose that, at least at Severalls, considerable efforts would be made to improve the social environment. Further surveys were therefore undertaken which showed that poverty of the social milieu had decreased, at all three hospitals, by 1964, and that the clinical condition of the patients had improved concomitantly, as we describe in Chapter 6. Even more significantly, there was a clear difference between patients whose social surroundings became socially richer, who tended to show fewer negative symptoms, and those whose social environment remained impoverished, who tended not to improve. Changes in drug treatment could not explain these facts.

It is still possible to think of an alternative non-social hypothesis for these results. There is a long-established clinical theory that the schizophrenic process gradually 'burns out'. It could therefore be argued that some patients eventually show improvement whatever their social environment. If so, they would be easier to resocialise, they could more easily be provided with clothes and other equipment, their contacts with the outside world would be easier to increase and the nurses' attitudes would naturally become more favourable. Hospitals where value is attached to making the social environment more stimulating would take advantage of such opportunities, but the social changes would be a *result*, and not a *cause*, of the clinical improvement. This would account for the results given in Chapter 6.

The major difficulty about accepting this explanation as it stands is that the clinical poverty syndrome was most marked in 1960, when patients had been in hospital, on average, sixteen years, and should have had plenty of time to improve if they were going to do so. However, there is a way of putting both hypotheses to the test since, if the social environment should, for any reason, become socially *more* impoverished, the predictions are quite different. On the burning-out hypothesis, clinical improvement will continue anyway, since it is not dependent on the social milieu. On the social hypothesis, there should be clinical deterioration.

We showed in Chapter 7 that there was indeed a reversal of fortunes at Netherne and Mapperley, where the social conditions, after an initial improvement, returned to approximately their previous level. At both hospitals the process of clinical improvement was also reversed, and patients became more socially withdrawn. One cannot suppose that the curves representing social and clinical change, in Figure 7.21 (p. 237), which move in phase with each other, but which show concomitant improvement and deterioration at different times in different hospitals, are describing the natural history of an illness.

The hypothesis that the social conditions under which a patient lives (particularly poverty of the social environment) are actually responsible for part of the symptomatology (particularly the negative symptoms), has been subjected to a number of fairly rigorous tests, any one of which it might well have failed, but it has not been disproved. In the remainder of this chapter it will be assumed to be correct.

THE EFFECT OF THE SOCIAL ENVIRONMENT ON FLORID
SYMPTOMS

In long-stay patients, florid symptoms such as delusions, incoherence of speech and socially embarrassing behaviour are much less in evidence than poverty of speech or social withdrawal. This may be because protection from the stresses of everyday life removes the precipitants of such symptoms, it may be due to medication, or it may be part of the natural history of schizophrenia (our own preference would be for the first of these alternatives). Incoherence of speech showed some improvement over the years, but less than the other symptoms studied. On the other hand, coherently-expressed delusions tended to improve more often than other symptoms. There was no evidence that florid symptoms increased with social stimulation, but the process of social improvement may well have been gradual enough to prevent this. However, it could have occurred and then been counteracted without leaving any impact on our measurements. The evidence that rehabilitation procedures may precipitate relapse of florid symptoms is very suggestive and the possibility is certainly not ruled out by our findings.

Patients with coherently-expressed delusions are less likely than others to be very long-stay. Their symptomatology is not related to social and clinical poverty (if anything, the reverse) and they do not have institutional attitudes to anything like the same extent. They do have unrealistic attitudes, however. It is clear that this is a separate group of schizophrenic patients, with a much higher (though often an idiosyncratic) motivation, and not so vulnerable to develop institutionalism. Venables' work confirms this view.

Patients with severe incoherence of speech are much more equivalent to those with severe negative symptoms, and their response to social changes seemed to follow similar patterns.

THE RELATIONSHIP BETWEEN 'NEGATIVE' AND 'FLORID' SYMPTOMS

It is convenient to classify patients with coherently-expressed delusions as the predominant symptom in a separate group. The data for the remaining large majority are consistent with the hypothesis that thought disorder is usually present in chronic schizophrenic patients, who react by cutting down their communication with other people, thus showing the negative symptoms such as social withdrawal, blunting of affect and poverty of speech. This cannot be the complete explanation for related negative symptoms such as slowness and under-activity, though it could be contributory even here. In under-stimulating social surroundings this tendency is given full rein and tends to proceed too far. The patient may become completely pre-occupied with inner experiences such as hallucinations, or appear to have little inner life at all. In over-stimulating social surroundings, the patient is unable to withdraw into a protective shell, but forced to interact and communicate. Florid symptoms then manifest themselves more openly and the resulting speech and behaviour abnormalities lead to a 'crisis'.

Somewhere between these two extremes lies the optimum social environment, in which the behaviour and expectations of others are clearly evident, predictable and not too demanding (though also not too permissive). It is very characteristic, in these circumstances, for patients to say that they only hear voices at night when they go to bed or when they are not paying attention during the day.

Whether or not negative symptoms develop partly as a protective mechanism, they are clearly related to the basic process in schizophrenia. Venables showed that they were highly correlated with psycho-physiological variables and that the most withdrawn schizophrenic patient was the most 'over-aroused' according to his measures. An under-stimulating social environment therefore increases a *primary* impairment, social stimulation reduces it, and one can speak in the strictest sense of social treatment.

In addition, however, it seems probable (if only from the literary evidence mentioned in Chapter 1) that social withdrawal can develop in many people exposed for long years to a socially impoverished and restricted environment, whatever the reason for the original incarceration. That is, social withdrawal can be a 'secondary' impairment. It is pointless to try to separate primary from secondary components in schizophrenic withdrawal. The most important characteristic to remember is that the schizophrenic patient is *vulnerable* to an under-stimulating environment and is likely to react with a much larger degree of social withdrawal. This vulnerability remains even when the social milieu is favourable and withdrawal therefore reduced to a minimum. The extent of the vulnerability probably varies greatly and it may be negligible in some patients, but it would be unwise to assume that it is not present, since unfavourable environments may occur anywhere, not only in mental hospitals, and abolishing hospital institutionalism does not solve all the problems of schizophrenia.

HOW MUCH CLINICAL IMPROVEMENT WAS THERE?

It is clear from our results that the discharge of a long-stay patient from hospital does not necessarily indicate a recent clinical improvement. Of the 53 patients discharged during the seven-and-a-half years of the study, 23 left during the first four years. Nearly all these were only moderately impaired in 1960 and had then wished to leave. The other group of 30 patients contained many more who were severely disabled in 1960 but they improved measurably by 1964 and it was demonstrated that this clinical improvement was an important factor leading to discharge.

Apart from this, the extent of the improvement shown by our figures can only be gathered from the examples given in Chapter 8. Most of the clinical improvement was shown by a decrease in social withdrawal, flatness of affect and other negative symptoms, though florid symptoms (particularly coherently-expressed delusions) also improved somewhat. We calculated that about one-fifth of patients who were not discharged between 1960 and 1964 showed a fairly marked improvement, evident from their conversation as recorded at the time of interview. (Another 10 per cent showed less definite changes for the better.) This proportion might appear small but it should be seen in context. If social improvements had not been taking place at the hospitals the tendency would have been for the patients to become more withdrawn and reticent, simply with the passing of the years. That such deterioration was mainly prevented, and that so large a proportion as one-fifth of the patients actually improved, is a considerable achievement.

'SECONDARY' IMPAIRMENTS: ATTITUDES TO DISCHARGE

Attitude to discharge is not a pure measure of secondary factors, since patients who expressed coherent delusions were less likely to adopt unfavourable attitudes while patients with severe negative symptoms were more likely to be indifferent. Poverty of the social surroundings also had some influence. However, independently of these contributions, there was a strong relationship between attitude to discharge and length of stay. The longer a patient has been in hospital the more likely he or she is to wish to stay or to be indifferent about leaving. Thus the hypothesis derived from earlier work was confirmed.

Unfavourable attitudes were very resistant to change. The social improvements brought about at the three hospitals—particularly those at Severalls—did not seem to do more than slow down the process whereby patients tend to adopt a wish to remain in hospital as they stay longer. Previous work on changing attitudes to work outside hospital, in long-stay patients with schizophrenia, showed that the most successful technique is a realistic course of preparation which demonstrates to patients, relatives and staff that they do have the capability (Wing, Bennett and Denham, 1964). A planned system of travelling by public transport and other everyday activities, trial weekends and holidays with relatives or in hostels, is probably the best way to change attitudes to discharge in selected patients.

Of the 23 patients who were discharged by the time of the second survey in 1964, 19 had had favourable attitudes when seen in 1960. Of the remaining 30 patients, who were outside hospital at the time of the final survey in January 1968, only 12 had wanted to leave in 1960, and a further 5 did so at the time of the latest survey before leaving. Thus 13 patients either changed their minds later on, or were still doubtful when they did leave.

THE NATURE OF INSTITUTIONALISM IN MENTAL HOSPITALS

Indifference about leaving lies at the very heart of institutionalism, and we would expect to find it developing in the inmates of most total institutions, particularly in those from vulnerable groups such as the physically handicapped, mentally retarded or those with inadequate personalities. Schizophrenic patients are probably particularly at risk because of their vulnerability to social under-stimulation, which also contributes to the development of unfavourable attitudes. In long-stay patients, these elements—clinical and social poverty and 'institutionalism'—often occur together and it may then seem difficult to disentangle the elements. However, secondary impairment develops in patients who have only mild or moderate clinical symptoms the longer they stay in hospital. It is important to consider the primary and secondary disabilities separately because the treatments are different. We have seen that an increase in activity, which reduces social withdrawal and affective blunting, does not necessarily change attitudes. On the other hand, more personal possessions, a smarter hairstyle, and so on, do not necessarily lead to clinical change, though they would be expected to reduce secondary impairments. In severely-handicapped patients the first task is to bring about clinical improvement—but preventive work, to prevent deterioration in self-respect and self-confidence and to stop the development of institutionalised attitudes, is also needed. In moderately-handicapped patients the main task is to change attitudes, or to prevent them from becoming unfavourable.

Thus institutionalism in mental hospitals should be regarded as no different, in principle, from the condition that develops in other institutions, although it may be seen in its most severe form in long-stay schizophrenic patients.

The organisation of social therapy in mental hospitals

The second part of this discussion will be devoted to a consideration of how the knowledge about social methods of treatment gained in this study may be applied. The first question to decide is which changes in social environment were most important in bringing about the clinical improvement.

WHICH SOCIAL CHANGES WERE MOST IMPORTANT?

The analysis presented in Chapter 6 brings out quite clearly that the most important single factor associated with improvement of primary handicaps was a reduction in the amount of time doing nothing. There was a general improvement in the social environment of all patients, but it was much greater for those who were better clinically in 1964 and, above all, the amount of inactivity had markedly decreased. Table 6.14 (p. 223) shows what kinds of activities took the place of idleness. The only really important category distinguishing patients who improved clinically from those who did not was 'work and occupational therapy'. Although time spent watching television or listening to the radio or in various leisure occupations (a very diverse category) also increased, there was little to choose between the increase in patients who improved clinically and the increase in those who did not. More time was spent watching television or listening to the radio or in various leisure pursuits (knitting, talking, going for walks, etc.) by those who improved clinically *and* by those who did not. It was probably the introduction of industrial work at Severalls which accounted for much of the clinical improvement there. Thus inactivity appears to be one of the greatest dangers for the chronic schizophrenic patient and seems to be directly responsible for a certain proportion of clinical symptomatology such as flatness of affect, poverty of speech and social withdrawal.

However, ward restrictiveness also seems to play an independent part in promoting or maintaining negative symptoms. This may well be because a highly restrictive ward is under-stimulating even when patients are engaged in doing something—their activities are of a more habitual and less interesting kind.

The other social changes, such as increased contact with the outside world, a more optimistic mood among the nursing staff and an increased supply of personal belongings, are less important so far as primary disabilities are concerned. They are nevertheless of major importance in reducing secondary handicaps. A woman with well-fitting clothes, pleasantly styled hair and judiciously applied make-up, who spends most of her day working as a typist in the nurses' training school, who makes expeditions to the local shops when she wishes to and patronises the town cinema with her friend, is far removed from the stereotype of the 'back ward' schizophrenic; and the attitudes of staff and relatives, as well as her own attitudes to herself, depend in large measure on this 'front' that she is able to show to the world. The same patient, in Kerry Ward in 1960, presented quite a different image, one which would have confirmed the gloomy views which used to be common currency among those who thought they knew about the course of schizophrenia.

Clearly, these changes have to be brought about gradually; and, when there are limited resources, certain patients will receive attention at the expense of others. Thus, at Severalls, the restrictiveness of the ward regimes did not decrease very remarkably overall although the social conditions in the wards, and the social experiences of many patients, did improve considerably. Similarly, in the American hospital, there was very high restrictiveness combined with relatively low morbidity. The creation of a liberal regime in which the patients could participate fully according to their ability is, however, an important step in their resocialisation and a more economical way of achieving part of it. The major lesson to be drawn is that general social changes are no substitute for specific social treatment aimed at each individual, and based upon a detailed knowledge of his handicaps. The two approaches are complementary.

We did not attempt to measure self-attitudes in patients in this series, but we would certainly suggest that they improved, in so far as they reflected the new social status that many people were able to attain. They were, however, still in hospital, and more specific measures to change the whole atmosphere away from that of an institution towards those of commoner social groupings—in particular the family—had not proceeded very far except at Netherne (and, even there, only for a small proportion of the patients in our series). These were traditional environments, removing many of those elements which had disfigured them in the custodial era, but not radically reforming their social structures. One would not expect profound changes in attitudes to discharge or to work, under these circumstances. Whether it is reasonable to expect further substantial changes in our mental hospitals, or whether the peak of benevolence and informed stimulation which we found at Netherne is the best that can be achieved, we will discuss in the final section. Meanwhile, since most hospitals have not yet reached the standards of Netherne, a more practical question may be formulated—how is it done?

THE ORGANISATION NECESSARY TO BRING ABOUT CLINICAL IMPROVEMENT

None of the three hospitals we studied claimed to be a 'therapeutic community' in the sense described by Jones (1968) or Clark (1964). Several of the wards at Netherne did have regular patient–staff meetings, and patients were organised in small groups, each with its own nurse or occupational therapist. There was certainly an emphasis on communication between staff at different levels of the various hierarchies. On the other hand, the group organisation was not as thoroughgoing, the staff 'democratisation' was not as far-reaching, the communication links were not as ubiquitous, the work organisation was not as 'creative', the leadership pattern was not as ill-defined and the staff routine not as 'spontaneous' as the requirements laid down would require—nor, in any case, would these have been regarded as ideal, at Netherne.

Nevertheless, in the sense that the social conditions provided certainly minimised morbidity to a point lower than in the other two hospitals, the term 'therapeutic community' can be used to describe Netherne in the practical, as opposed to the theoretical, sense. Treatment was being applied by means of manipulating the social environment and, even if it could have been taken further, it is difficult to think of a hospital, whatever its philosophy, where an equivalent demonstration has been made. The emphasis on industrial work, as a means of achieving a neutral stimulus to which the patient can respond without over-involvement, and risk of reactivating florid symptoms, is clearly justified. Dr Freudenberg has shown, in Chapter 3, that Netherne had passed through the same historical phases as Severalls, before 1960, and we have little doubt that the relative excellence of its social environment was responsible for the lower morbidity in the patients there.

The organisation of the patient's day in Longfield Villa, described in Chapter 8, may be taken as the model towards which all three hospitals were striving and which Netherne came closest to attaining. Ideally, patients should do things for themselves; get up, get their meals, do the chores, go to work, spend their leisure time and organise their way of life, as they would if they were not in hospital and not handicapped. This means a constant testing to see whether the time has come for a particular function to be actively taken over by a patient rather than being passively exercised by a helper. Left to himself, the severely-handicapped schizophrenic patient lapses into inactivity. With active supervision this tendency is counteracted—but for how long need the active supervision be kept up? When can it be relaxed? These are some of the essential questions of social treatment (Wing and Freudenberg, 1961) and they may be more easily answered if staff and patients can share experiences in regular group sessions.

Barton (1959) in his booklet on 'Institutional Neurosis' gives instructions for countering the tendency towards institutionalism. The suggestions are clear-cut and didactic and, again, there is little emphasis on groups in Maxwell Jones' sense. We can only remark that Barton's methods are successful (particularly the reduction of 'enforced idleness') in so far as they can be applied without extra trained staff, and that, since they represent the distilled wisdom of a whole generation of psychiatrists looking at the problems of mental hospitals with new eyes, they ought by now to have been widely adopted. Both Barton and Freudenberg emphasise the fundamental importance of staff morale, and at this point they join forces with the proponents of the 'therapeutic community' concept. However, a major purpose of achieving high morale in the treatment teams was to ensure that specific procedures for helping schizophrenic patients were applied with the greatest efficiency.

Underlying the policy at all three hospitals was the assumption that specialised environments should be created for various categories of patient. Thus Longfield Villa was set up for the most severely handicapped patients, while Downswood catered for patients who were able to participate in life outside hospital to a certain extent and for whom there was a fair prospect of discharge in the relatively near

future. At Mapperley there were wards run by the patients themselves, with only an experienced part-time staff member to keep an
eye on things. At Netherne there was a range of industrial workshops
catering for patients with different levels of handicap. Early (1965)
advocated 'ladders' of domestic and vocational rehabilitation with
sufficient rungs on each (that is, with a sufficient variety of social
environments) to accommodate all the patients, both within and
outside hospital, who need help. Netherne provided the greatest
variety of environments within the hospital, but both Mapperley
and Severalls adopted the principle.

Thus from the intimate level of the ward nurse or occupational
therapist, engaged in helping a schizophrenic patient to function in a
social environment, to the more distant level of hospital planning
of specialised workshops and wards, the intention was to provide
specific treatment for specific individuals.

Why then, did more patients not improve? More important, why
did the final survey in January 1968 show such a disappointing
fall-off, and even reversal, in the rate of improvement?

WHY DID SOCIAL CONDITIONS NOT IMPROVE MORE, AND IS
REFORM NECESSARILY SHORT-LIVED?

It should first of all be emphasised that the fall-off at Mapperley and
Netherne was only to the 1960 level—the much larger improvements
which must have taken place before 1960 were not affected.

About half of the patients who were severely impaired in 1960
remained in much the same condition in 1964. Basically, as we have
already shown, this may have been because their social surroundings
had not been measurably changed. Forty-nine out of 78 severely
impaired patients who did not improve clinically between 1960 and
1964, also showed no decrease in amount of time doing nothing. It
may be assumed that some of them would have improved if they had
been given a more socially stimulating environment. (The 29 who did
not improve clinically, even though they *were* activated, might have
required more time before they responded, or they might have been
incapable of response.) It is an old adage in mental hospital practice
that one should never give up hope in schizophrenia. Any patient,
however seemingly intractable the condition, retains the capacity to
surprise the persistent therapist.

One reason why the social improvements were not more widespread seems to be that all the increase in activation was obtained by a redeployment of the same (or possibly even fewer) staff, and that there was a physical limit to what could be done. At Severalls, for example, we had the impression that extra work with one handicapped patient—the kind of persistent activation that slowly and gradually brings its accumulation of small rewards until something like a major change is eventually seen—could sometimes only be carried out at the expense of neglecting someone else. This may be the explanation of the fact that some moderately-handicapped patients at Severalls, who perhaps seemed to require less attention than others, were actually allowed to become less active and therefore more withdrawn (see Figure 7.25, p. 241). A consideration of the number of hours work involved shows how feasible this explanation is. Even if a productivity expert could demonstrate how to resocialise patients with the minimum waste of staff power, there would be insufficient facilities to do everything that a keen social psychiatrist would feel to be necessary.

The problem becomes more complicated when one considers the unequivocal evidence of Figure 7.21, p. 237. It is true that other patients might have benefited during the early years of the study, if more resources had been available. However, during the later years, progress actually began to fall off. The main change at Mapperley, for example, took place between 1960 and 1962 but, by 1964, things had begun to slip back again and, by 1968, there was little difference from the original situation. This conclusion paints too pessimistic a picture because it does not give credit for the number of patients discharged or attending as day patients. It does show, however, how difficult it is to *maintain* social innovations. Even at Netherne, although the social conditions, and the patients, retained their original advantageous position relative to the other hospitals, the improvement demonstrated between 1960 and 1964 had largely dissipated by 1968. Again, the discharged patients are not taken into account and the residual population obviously presents particularly difficult problems—but to lose hard-won gains is disappointing. The process can be studied in slow motion, as it were, at Severalls where there was most room for change and where improvement was most striking. Again twenty-six patients who were discharged have been omitted. But the remaining group showed marked progress between 1960 and 1962, slightly less but still sizeable improvement between 1962 and 1964 and then a much slower rate of change until 1968 (except for outside contact which is still going ahead). In 1968 the patients were beginning to be rather more withdrawn, on average, although still very much more sociable and active than in 1960.

Three kinds of explanation suggest themselves. One might invoke the effect of age, though this seems to have been a variable with surprisingly little significance throughout the analysis. Perhaps, as the patient approaches 60, even the keenest and most sensitive of therapists begins to feel that other patients have a higher claim for attention. It is impossible to rule out this explanation altogether, but it can hardly account for the whole trend. Figure 7.24 (p. 241) shows that the same trends are occurring in patients under 45 years of age. Even in 1968, more than half the remaining patients were under 60 and one-third were under 50. The second kind of explanation is, in some ways, more disheartening; that the therapists (doctors, nurses, occupational therapists and supervisors) began to feel, at different turning-points in different hospitals, that they had done as much as they could; that expenditure of further time and energy would prejudice the chances of other patients, or simply that enough was enough. The fact that Dr Macmillan retired in 1966, that Dr Freudenberg was seconded to the Ministry of Health from 1961 to 1964, and that Dr D. H. Bennett, who had done so much to build up the rehabilitation and resettlement services at Netherne, left in June 1962, must also be taken into account.

A further consideration which must be discussed, since it will certainly occur to our readers, is whether the presence of a research team at the hospitals in 1960, and the knowledge that they would return two years later, had anything to do with the early improvements. We did inform the three superintendents of the 1960 results, but there was no way of checking whether extra action was taken to influence the results of the second survey which would not have occurred anyway. On the other hand, we did not decide to undertake the 1964 surveys until shortly before approaching the hospitals again and the same is true of the final collection of data in January 1968, so that we are fairly sure that prior knowledge of these surveys can have had little effect on the results.

Perhaps the explanation that will most readily occur to those familiar with present-day mental hospitals is the simple one that priorities have changed. With the full flowering of the early discharge policy, with admissions and re-admissions continuing to mount, with out-patient, day patient, domiciliary and consultative services all presenting steadily increasing demands, with psycho-geriatric work taking up a larger and larger proportion of clinical time, the attention that doctors can give to long-stay patients, and the number of staff who can be spared for rehabilitation, must inevitably diminish. This consideration brings up the whole question of the future of the mental hospital.

The future of the mental hospital

To some psychiatrists, this book must seem an anachronism, reviving echoes of forgotten problems. To them, the long-stay question is solved. Once the present, steadily decreasing, number of long-stay patients has finally disappeared, the new accumulation will be negligible. Chronic schizophrenia can be prevented by drugs, or by family therapy, or by a combination of various community treatments, and the long-stay patient will be relegated to psychiatric history.

It is too soon to evaluate all the complicated and sometimes contradictory trends which can be discerned in recent statistics, though it is clear that long-stay schizophrenics are still with us. If we return, however, to the point we made in Chapter 1, that psychiatric services should be evaluated in terms of their effect on the morbidity of patients and relatives, one can put together a tentative story and draw some tentative conclusions. We studied 111 schizophrenic patients first admitted to Mapperley, Netherne and Severalls hospitals in 1956 (Brown *et al.*, 1966). Five years after first admission just over one-quarter of them were still severely handicapped, although only 14 were actually in hospital. The burden on relatives and the community caused by the severely impaired patients was rarely negligible, and in some cases it was intolerable. Very few patients indeed had been given the benefit of rehabilitation services. We thought that the process of accumulation of secondary handicaps had continued, even though most of the patients had not become institutionalised in the narrow sense of the term. Further studies are currently being carried out to discover how far rehabilitation methods which were worked out for 'long-stay' patients (Wing, Bennett and Denham, 1964) are applicable to the new kind of 'long-term' patients now presenting. It is quite possible to ignore such problems—relatives often do not complain and the reputation of mental hospitals has been such that prolonged residence in them is still regarded with horror. But as Early (1965) points out, the ladders of domestic and industrial rehabilitation can only be climbed to the top by a proportion of patients—others will get so far and then need settlement at that level. The function of asylum, of protection from the ordinary stresses of everyday life, may still be required for some (Catterson, Bennett and Freudenberg, 1963). Others may need sheltered workshops and/or sheltered living arrangements. The expertise of mental hospital staff is still required and it seems probable that many mental hospitals will evolve further, in order to undertake the rehabilitation functions for a community, as well as providing treatment and asylum.

Whatever services are found to be necessary, for whatever numbers, we think that the experience of these three hospitals in dealing with one of the most intractable problems in psychiatry will remain valid and should not be ignored. Not only can it be demonstrated that the social treatments carried out by mental hospital staff do have value and that the course of schizophrenic illnesses can be influenced in hospital, as it can outside, but there is a salutary reminder that efforts must be kept up and that reform itself has a natural history. This demonstration has lessons and a warning for social psychiatrists who are directing, as they must, much of their attention to problems outside hospital. New forms of community agency must be developed in which the best aspects of the mental hospital tradition are preserved even if the buildings themselves are not. The services provided by the various specialised social environments of the good mental hospital are still needed. The experience of the rehabilitation team is relevant to the new problems of community psychiatry. If these skills and traditions are lost it will be a long time before they are developed again. Rehabilitation remains one of the most necessary, as well as one of the most rewarding, aspects of psychiatry, and its scientific basis is beginning to unite biological, psychological and social researches in a way which may prove a model for other fields of medicine. The present ferment of change provides an opportunity for further progress but only if the lessons of the past—particularly the state of 'community care' which preceded the foundation of the early hospitals for 'moral treatment'—are remembered and profitably used.

TABLES AND FIGURES

TABLE 2.1. *Distribution of schizophrenic patients in six categories of 'present mental state'*

	Clinical category	Stone House, 1964 (both sexes)			Netherne, 1960 (both sexes)			Three hospitals 1960 (females only)		
		N	%	Mean S.W. score	N	%	Mean S.W. score	N	%	Mean S.W. score
1a and 1b	Moderate symptoms only	16	20	1·8	45	30	1·4	77	28	1·5
1c	Moderate speech symptoms but severe flatness of affect	27	34	3·0	22	15	4·2	15	5	3·4
2	Coherent delusions predominant	13	17	3·0	28	19	2·4	29	11	2·4
3	Incoherence of speech predominant	16	20	5·8	15	10	4·4	42	15	4·5
4	Poverty of speech predominant	2	3	6·0	30	20	4·3	70	26	5·3
5	Mute or almost mute	5	6	10·4	10	7	9·6	40	15	10·1
	Total	79	100		150	101		273	100	

TABLE 2.2. *Means, standard deviations, maximum score possible and range of actual scores on certain variables in 1960* (N = 273) *and correlation between 1960 and 1964 scores* (N = 233).

(Three hospitals)

1960	Mean	Standard deviation	Maximum possible score	Range of actual scores	Correlation 1960–1964
S.W.	4·62	4·13	16	0–15	0·66
S.E.	1·64	1·80	8	0–7	0·29
Occupation	4·68	3·28	15	0–15	0·44
Outside contact	5·34	4·18	15	0–15	0·70
Phenothiazine	2·33	2·39	—*	0–12	0·38
Nurses' attitudes	6·78	3·84	13	0–13	0·59
Possessions	21.49	16·39	70	0–63	0·62
Hours doing nothing	4·48	3·39	10·75**	0–10·75	0·44

* The highest dose actually administered was equivalent to 1,200 mg. of Chlorpromazine (i.e. 12 units).
** On average, patients spent 10·85 hours in bed and 2·40 hours at table or at toilet. The time available for 'doing anything' was therefore 10·75 hours on average.

TABLE 3.1. *Employment and unemployment at Netherne, 1962*
(Total number of patients, 1,792)

	Men				Women			
	Under 60	%	Over 60	%	Under 60	%	Over 60	%
Residing in hospital, working outside	34	**8·7**	5	**3·0**	49	**8·1**	3	**0·5**
Industrial subcontracts in hospital	154	**39·3**	14	**8·3**	210	**34·8**	20	**3·2**
Utility work in hospital	137	**34·9**	60	**35·5**	140	**23·2**	49	**7·8**
Domestic work in hospital	14	**3·8**	18	**10·7**	57	**9·5**	99	**15·8**
Total remunerative employment	339	**86·7**	97	**57·5**	456	**75·6**	171	**27·3**
Unemployed and unoccupied	22	**5·6**	60	**35·5**	86	**14·3**	224	**35·7**
Number of patients O.T. unpaid	31	**7·9**	12	**7·1**	61	**10·1**	233	**37·1**
Total patients unemployed	53	**13·5**	72	**42·6**	147	**24·4**	457	**72·8**
Total employed and unemployed	392	**100·2**	169	**100·1**	603	**100·0**	628	**100·1**

TABLE 3.2. (a) *Employment and unemployment at Netherne, 1965*
(Total number of patients, 1,743)

	Men				Women			
	Under 60	%	Over 60	%	Under 60	%	Over 60	%
Residing in hospital, working outside	48	12·4	3	1·9	62	10·9	5	0·8
Industrial subcontracts in hospital	116	30·0	18	11·6	134	23·6	26	4·1
Utility work in hospital	125	32·2	33	21·0	103	18·1	64	10·0
Domestic work in hospital	21	5·4	24	15·3	86	15·1	110	17·4
Total remunerative employment	310	80·0	78	49·8	385	67·7	205	32·3
Unemployed and un-occupied*	26	6·7	39	25·0	60	10·6	210	33·4
Number of patients O.T. unpaid	51	13·3	40	25·2	123	21·7	216	34·3
Total patients un-employed	77	20·0	79	50·2	183	32·3	426	67·7
Total employed and unemployed	387	100	157	100	568	100	631	100

Tables 3.2(a)–(c) are from Freudenberg, 1967.
* In the unemployed group, recent admissions and patients aged 60 and over predominate. At present 788 patients are aged 60 and over.

TABLE 3.2 (b). *Patients working in the community while remaining resident in the hospital (night patients)*

Men		Women	
*Industrial rehabilitation unit	1	Industrial rehabilitation unit	—
**Industrial therapy organization	9	Industrial therapy organization	5
***Sheltered employment	4	Sheltered employment	2
****Open employment	38	Open employment	60
Total	52	Total	67

* Assessment unit for 100 disabled workers, physical and psychiatric, run by Ministry of Labour. (Duration of training 8 weeks.)
** Private non-profit-making organisation, subsidised by Ministry of Labour for rehabilitation of psychiatric patients. (Duration of training six months —one-year stay.)
*** Private non-profit-making company, subsidised by Ministry of Labour for permanent employment of disabled patients.
**** Open competitive employment.

TABLE 3.2(*c*). *Patients classified according to payments received*

Industrial payments of total employed			
Up to 5*s*.	6*s*.–10*s*.	11*s*.–20*s*.	21*s*.+
24·1 %	17·8 %	37·1 %	11·0 %

TABLE 3.3. *Employment and unemployment at Netherne, 1968*
(Total number of patients, 1,533)

	Men				Women			
	Under 60	%	Over 60	%	Under 60	%	Over 60	%
Residing in hospital, working outside	42	12·3	3	1·7	51	12·5	6	1·0
Industrial subcontracts in hospital	126	36·9	18	10·1	99	24·3	21	3·5
Utility work in hospital	80	23·4	47	26·4	86	21·1	56	9·3
Domestic work in hospital	26	7·6	16	9·0	45	11·0	96	15·9
Total remunerative employment	274	80·2	84	47·2	281	68·9	179	29·7
Unemployed and un-occupied	38	11·1	51	28·7	58	14·2	220	36·4
Number of patients O.T. unpaid	30	8·8	43	24·3	69	16·9	206	34·0
Total patients un-employed	68	19·9	94	52·9	127	31·1	426	70·4
Total employed and unemployed	342	100·1	178	100·1	408	100·0	605	100·1

TABLE 4.1. Intercorrelations between certain social and clinical variables, 1960

(Three hospitals; N = 273)

	1	2	3	4	5	6	7	8	9	10	11	12	13	14	15
1. Outside contact	1·000														
2. Favourable nurses' attitudes	0·578	1·000													
3. Personal possessions	0·557	0·704	1·000												
4. Occupation	0·426	0·630	0·641	1·000											
5. Time doing nothing	−0·509	−0·684	−0·653	−0·637	1·000										
6. Social withdrawal	−0·481	−0·655	−0·564	−0·468	0·634	1·000									
7. Flatness of affect	−0·468	−0·572	−0·552	−0·410	0·538	0·601	1·000								
8. Poverty of speech	−0·344	−0·451	−0·519	−0·315	0·464	0·550	0·699	1·000							
9. Incoherence of speech	−0·180	−0·172	−0·126	−0·088	0·208	0·030	0·212	−0·156	1·000						
10. Coherently-expressed delusions	0·141	0·278	0·302	0·255	−0·210	−0·261	−0·132	−0·355	0·235	1·000					
11. Socially embarrassing behaviour	−0·199	−0·360	−0·207	−0·207	0·249	0·291	0·329	0·195	0·207	0·012	1·000				
12. Length of stay	−0·322	−0·334	−0·279	−0·232	0·158	0·302	0·253	0·268	0·073	−0·249	0·123	1·000			
13. Age	−0·156	−0·063	−0·098	−0·127	0·050	0·026	−0·003	−0·101	0·198	0·110	−0·003	0·447	1·000		
14. Dose of phenothiazine	0·117	−0·037	0·079	−0·047	−0·084	0·003	−0·002	−0·044	−0·118	0·024	0·150	−0·040	−0·211	1·000	
15. Unfavourable attitude to discharge	−0·374	−0·385	−0·337	−0·290	0·338	0·402	0·447	0·278	0·248	−0·219	0·153	0·386	0·182	−0·119	1·000

(Significance levels for N = 100; r = 0·195, p < 0·05; r = 0·254, p < 0·01; r = 0·32, p < 0·001.)

TABLE 4.2. Intercorrelations between certain social and clinical variables, 1964

(Three hospitals; N = 233)

	1	2	3	4	5	6	7	8	9	10	11	12	13	14	15
1. Outside contact	1·000														
2. Favourable nurses' attitudes	0·507	1·000													
3. Personal possessions	0·526	0·613	1·000												
4. Occupation	0·334	0·507	0·471	1·000											
5. Time doing nothing	-0·405	-0·688	-0·486	-0·510	1·000										
6. Social withdrawal	-0·486	-0·719	-0·542	-0·385	0·703	1·000									
7. Flatness of affect	-0·501	-0·636	-0·521	-0·376	0·494	0·605	1·000								
8. Poverty of speech	-0·476	-0·648	-0·543	-0·272	0·472	0·603	0·731	1·000							
9. Incoherence of speech	-0·140	-0·081	-0·006	-0·085	0·130	0·105	0·259	0·030	1·000						
10. Coherently-expressed delusions	-0·040	0·147	0·162	0·079	-0·077	-0·171	0·008	-0·186	0·228	1·000					
11. Socially embarrassing behaviour	-0·049	-0·252	-0·215	-0·101	0·177	0·282	0·292	0·292	0·168	0·010	1·000				
12. Length of stay	-0·340	-0·262	-0·301	0·188	0·131	0·193	0·292	0·346	0·023	-0·168	-0·086	1·000			
13. Age	-0·239	-0·109	-0·148	-0·161	0·129	0·036	-0·038	-0·006	0·167	0·046	-0·235	0·440	1·000		
14. Dose of phenothiazine	0·121	-0·076	-0·042	0·010	-0·045	-0·047	-0·011	-0·033	-0·103	0·044	0·306	-0·709	-0·244	1·000	
15. Unfavourable attitude to discharge	-0·220	-0·229	-0·215	-0·171	0·172	0·249	0·323	0·293	0·281	-0·143	0·125	0·247	0·206	-0·081	1·000

(Significance levels for N = 100; r = 0·195, p < 0·05; r = 0·254, p < 0·01; r = 0·32, p < 0·001.)

Figure 4.3 201

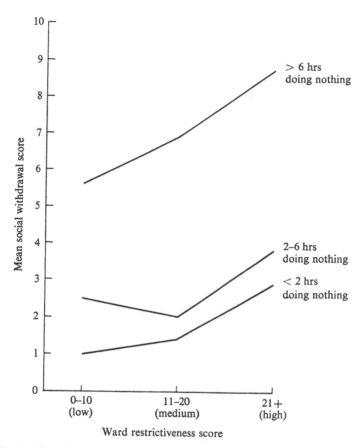

Fig. 4.3. Relationship between ward restrictiveness, hours doing nothing and social withdrawal, 1960. (Three hospitals; N = 273.)

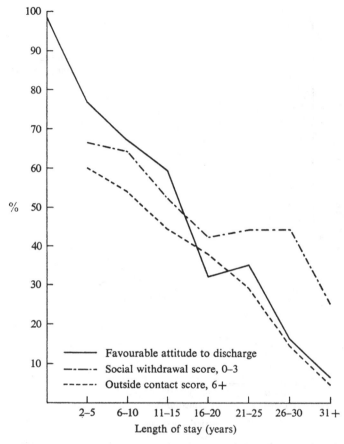

Fig. 4.4. Social withdrawal, attitude to discharge and outside contact, by length of stay, 1960. (Three hospitals; N = 273, except for under-two-year group—see text.)

Table 4.5–Figure 4.6 203

TABLE 4.5. *Attitude to discharge, by length of stay, 1960*

(Three hospitals; N = 273)

Attitude to discharge	Length of stay (years)			Total
	2–10	11–20	21+	
Wishes to leave	33	13	6	52
Ambivalent or vague	23	23	6	52
Indifferent	4	12	12	28
Wishes to stay	18	31	29	78
Total	78	79	53	210
Excluded because of muteness	6	15	16	37
Excluded because of incoherence	10	8	8	26
Grand total	94	102	77	273

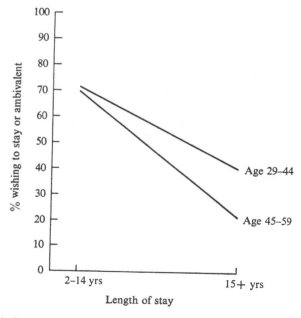

Fig. 4.6. Attitude to discharge, by length of stay and age, 1960. (Three hospitals; N = 210. Sixty-three mute and incoherent patients omitted.)

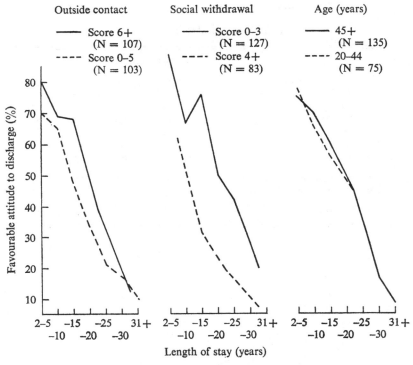

Fig. 4.7. Attitude to discharge by length of stay, outside contact, social withdrawal and age, 1960. (Three hospitals; N = 273.)

TABLE 4.8. *Favourable attitude to discharge and length of stay, 1960, when three social variables and two clinical variables are controlled*

(Three hospitals; N = 210. Sixty-three patients omitted because of muteness or incoherence of speech)

| Controlling variable | Length of stay (years) | | | | | |
| | 2–10 | | 11–20 | | 21+ | |
	N	%	N	%	N	%
Occupation score:						
6+	48	**77**	35	**51**	20	**15**
0–5	30	**63**	44	**41**	33	**27**
Favourable nurses' attitudes:						
8+	58	**79**	45	**56**	22	**23**
0–7	20	**50**	34	**32**	31	**23**
Time doing nothing (hours):						
0–3	53	**76**	34	**56**	26	**27**
> 3	25	**64**	45	**38**	27	**19**
Flatness of affect:						
1–3	44	**82**	38	**63**	19	**26**
4, 5	34	**59**	41	**29**	34	**21**
Poverty of speech:						
1–3	60	**77**	50	**60**	25	**28**
4, 5	18	**56**	29	**21**	28	**18**

TABLE 4.9. *Attitude to discharge: by clinical category, 1960*

(Three hospitals; N = 273)

	Clinical category	Wish to leave	Ambi-valent	Indif-ferent	Wish to stay	Excluded	Total
1	Moderate symptoms only	27	30	3	37	0	97
2	Coherent delusions predominant	12	11	1	4	1	29
3	Incoherence of speech predominant	3	1	5	9	24	42
4	Poverty of speech predominant	10	10	17	28	1	66
5	Mute or almost mute	0	0	2	0	37	39
	Total	52	52	28	78	63	273

TABLE 5.1. *Age of patients, 1960*

(Three hospitals separately; N = 273)

Age (years)	Netherne	Mapperley	Severalls
20–40	30	**18**	26
41–50	35	**29**	30
51–60	35	**53**	44
Total	100	**100***	100

* Per cent of 73.

($\chi^2 = 6 \cdot 40$, df = 4, p > 0·10.)

TABLE 5.2. *Length of stay of patients*

(Three hospitals separately; N = 273)

Length of stay (years)	Netherne	Mapperley	Severalls
2–10	42	**29**	30
11–20	38	**33**	40
21+	20	**38**	30
Total	100	**100***	100

* Per cent of 73.

($\chi^2 = 8 \cdot 62$, df = 4, p > 0·5.)

TABLE 5.3. *Occupation of patients' fathers, 1960*

(Three hospitals separately; N = 273)

	Netherne	Mapperley	Severalls
Professional and managerial	36	**14**	21
Lower administrative and clerical	8	**8**	16
Skilled manual	21	**16**	16
Semi-skilled manual	6	**21**	10
Unskilled manual	10	**18**	22
Not known	19	**23**	15
Total	100	**100***	100

* Per cent of 73.

TABLE 5.4. *Time budget of typical weekday, 1960*

(Three hospitals separately; N = 273)

	Netherne hours mins		Mapperley hours mins		Severalls hours mins	
On ward:						
Leisure activities	2	04	1	03	1	22
Ward work or occupational therapy	1	19	1	17	1	45
Toilet or meals	2	38	2	48	3	10
Nothing	2	40	2	40	5	36
Total on ward	8	41	7	48	11	53
Off ward:						
Occupational therapy or leisure	0	41	1	16	0	20
Work	3	32	2	50	0	47
Nothing	0	08	0	35	0	03
Total off ward	4	21	4	41	1	10
Total time out of bed	13	02	12	29	13	03

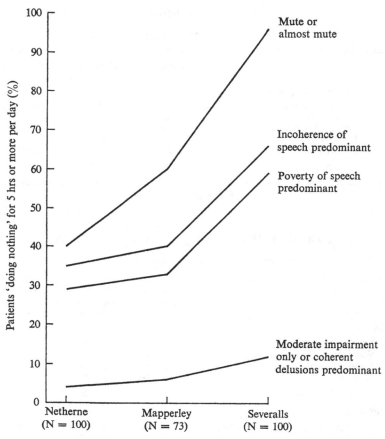

Fig. 5.5. Percentage of patients at the three hospitals who 'did nothing' for five hours a day or more in 1960: by clinical category. (Three hospitals separately; N = 273.)

Figure 5.6 209

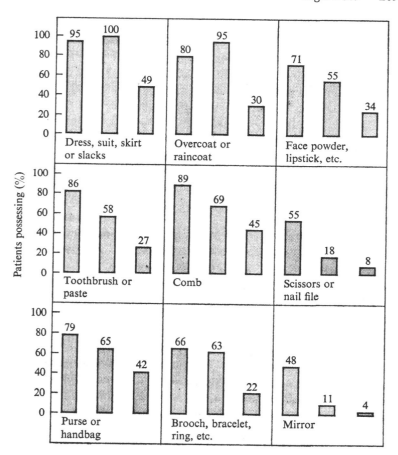

Fig. 5.6. Patients' personal possessions (supplied privately or by the hospital) in 1960. In each section the blocks represent Netherne (N = 100), Mapperley (N = 73) and Severalls (N = 100) in that order.

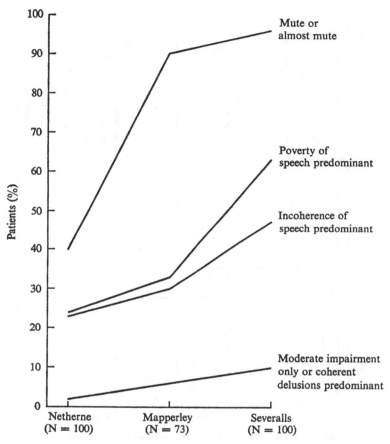

Fig. 5.7. Percentage of patients at the three hospitals who had no personal possessions apart from clothing and toilet articles in 1960: by clinical category. (Three hospitals separately; N = 273.)

Figure 5.8   211

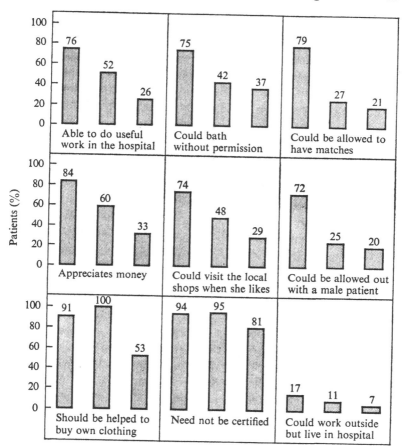

Fig. 5.8. Ward sisters' opinions about patients, 1960. In each section the blocks represent Netherne (N = 100), Mapperley (N = 73) and Severalls (N = 100) in that order.

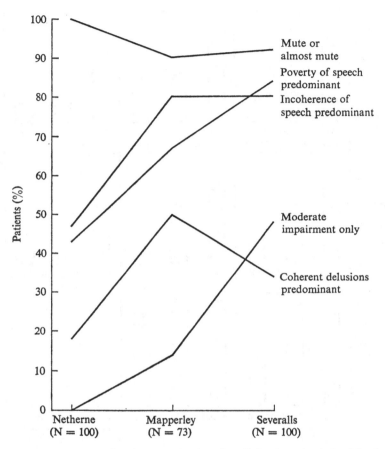

Fig. 5.9. Percentage of patients at the three hospitals who were judged by the ward sister to be incapable of useful work in the hospital in 1960: by clinical category. (Three hospitals separately; N = 273.)

TABLE 5.10. *Clinical classification of patients, 1960*

(Three hospitals separately; N = 273)

Clinical category	Netherne	Mapperley	Severalls
Moderately impaired:			
1a No florid symptoms, poverty of speech or flatness of affect	10 ⎫	15 ⎫	8 ⎫
1b Moderate symptoms only	21 ⎬ 40	19 ⎬ 39	13 ⎬ 23
1c Moderate speech symptoms but severe flatness of affect	9 ⎭	5 ⎭	2 ⎭
Severely ill:			
2 Coherent delusions predominant	17	8	6
3 Incoherence of speech predominant	17	14	15
4 Poverty of speech predominant	20 ⎫ 26	25 ⎫ 39	32 ⎫ 56
5 Mute or almost mute	6 ⎭	14 ⎭	24 ⎭
Total	100	100*	100

* Per cent of 73.
(Combining the moderately ill groups 1a, 1b and 1c:
$\chi^2 = 25\cdot81$, df = 8, p > 0·01.)

TABLE 5.11. *Clinical classification by occupation of patient's father, 1960*

(Three hospitals; N = 222)

Clinical category	Non-manual	Skilled manual	Semi-skilled manual	Un-skilled manual	Total
1 Moderate symptoms only	35	24	9	14	82
2 Coherent delusions predominant	13	5	3	3	24
3 Incoherence of speech predominant	11	7	6	4	28
4 Poverty of speech predominant	25	11	9	18	63
5 Mute or almost mute	13	2	4	6	25
Total	97	49	31	45	222*

($\chi^2 = 11\cdot92$, df = 12, p > 0·30.)
* In 51 cases the occupation of the father was not known.

TABLE 5.12. *Mean S.W. and S.E. scores by hospitals and by length of stay of patients, 1960*
(N = 273)

Length of stay (years)	Mean S.W. score				Mean S.E. score			
	Netherne	Mapperley	Severalls	Total	Netherne	Mapperley	Severalls	Total
2–10	2·2	2·6	3·9	2·9	1·0	1·7	1·5	1·3
11–20	2·8	4·5	6·1	4·5	1·3	2·3	1·3	1·5
21+	4·6	6·3	5·9	5·7	1·4	2·6	1·2	1·8
Total	3·0	4·6	5·5	4·3	1·2	2·3	1·3	1·5

TABLE 5.13. *Mean S.W. and S.E. scores by hospitals and occupation of patients' fathers*
(N = 273)

Hall-Jones occupational category	Mean S.W. score				Mean S.E. score			
	Netherne	Mapperley	Severalls	Total	Netherne	Mapperley	Severalls	Total
1, 2, 3 Professional, managerial	3·1	3·0	5·3	3·7	1·1	1·3	1·1	1·1
4, 5 Lower supervisory and clerical	4·1	3·8	5·3	4·7	3·0	2·0	1·8	2·1
6 Skilled manual	1·7	2·7	3·4	2·5	0·8	1·7	0·8	1·1
7 Semi-skilled manual	3·5	5·1	6·5	5·3	1·3	2·7	2·2	2·3
8 Unskilled manual	2·6	4·0	5·5	4·5	0·4	2·1	1·4	1·4
— Not known	3·4	7·5	6·9	5·7	1·4	3·3	1·1	1·7

TABLE 5.14. *Attitudes to discharge by hospitals and length of stay, 1960*
(N = 273)

Table 5.14 215

| Attitude to discharge | Length of stay (years) | | | | | | | | |
| | 2-10 | | | 11-20 | | | 21+ | | |
	Netherne	Mapperley	Severalls	Netherne	Mapperley	Severalls	Netherne	Mapperley	Severalls
Some desire to leave	14	6	12	9	4	6	3	1	—
Ambivalent	11	4	3	7	6	4	2	4	5
Indifferent	7	6	9	10	4	23	8	14	13
Desire to stay	10	5	6	12	10	7	7	9	12
Total	42	21	30	38	24	40	20	28	30

(Netherne: $\chi^2 = 6.88$, df = 2, p < 0.05
Mapperley: $\chi^2 = 5.60$, df = 2, p < 0.05
Severalls: $\chi^2 = 8.30$, df = 2, p < 0.05.)

TABLE 5.15. *Drugs prescribed for chronic schizophrenic patients in the three hospitals, 1960*
(N = 273)

	Size of 'unit'	Netherne 100 63		Mapperley 73 62		Severalls 100 70	
Number in sample Number receiving any day-time drug		N	Total daily 'units'	N	Total daily 'units'	N	Total daily 'units'
Chlorpromazine	100 mg.	23	44	33	76	44	94
Reserpine	1 mg.	13	47	18	57	—	—
Fentazine	4 mg.	—	—	7	22	4	14
Prochlorperazine	25 mg.	8	16	14	36	2	9
Trifluoperazine	10 mg.	24	42	1	1	7	8
Unnamed compound	50 mg.	—	—	—	—	10	20
Total 'units'		—	149	—	192*	—	145
Sodium amytal (by day)		5	20 gr.	16	109 gr.	8	60 gr.
Phenobarbitone (by day)		3	5 gr.	2	3 gr.	3	9 gr.
Sodium amytal (at night)		12	61 gr.	6	24 gr.	12	42 gr.

* 262 for 100 patients.

TABLE 6.1. *Improvement in 'poverty of the social environments' as measured by the mean scores on six variables in 1960 and 1964*

(Three hospitals; N = 233)

	Maximum score possible	Mean score in 1960	Mean score in 1964	Significance of difference (t-tests)
Outside contact	15	5·3	6·2	p < 0·001
Favourable nurses' attitudes	13	6·8	8·5	p < 0·001
Personal possessions	70	21·5	28·1	p < 0·001
Occupation	15	4·7	5·8	p < 0·001
Time doing nothing (hours)	—	4·5	3·5	p < 0·001
Ward restrictiveness*	50	23·5	17·0	p < 0·001

* Not based on the same patients. In 1960, N = 224. In 1964, N = 158.

TABLE 6.2. *Changes in nurses' attitudes, 1960–1964*

(Three hospitals; N = 233)

	% of patients		Mean improvement (%)
	1960	1964	
Could be on an open ward	94	100 ⎫	
Need not be certified	89	98 ⎬	+9·7
Could have own clothes	72	86 ⎭	
Knows the value of money	49	56 ⎫	
Could look after money	59	74 ⎪	
Could do useful work in hospital	55	70 ⎬	+13·8
Could go out to local shop	48	66 ⎭	
Could have scissors	41	64 ⎫	
Could bath alone	63	76 ⎪	
Could have matches	54	73 ⎬	+18·8
Could go out with men	39	59 ⎭	
Could work outside hospital now	11	18 ⎫	
Could be discharged now	8	8 ⎬	+3·5

TABLE 6.3. *Increase in personal possessions, 1960–1964*

(Three hospitals; N = 233)

	% owning		Mean improvements (%)
	1960	1964	
Dress or suit	79	98 ⎫	
Overcoat or raincoat	64	95 ⎬	+27·3
Brush, comb, etc.	66	98 ⎭	
Purse or handbag	59	80 ⎫	
Toothbrush	57	72 ⎪	
Make-up materials	51	67 ⎬	+17·3
Personal ornament	49	66 ⎭	
Mirror	30	37 ⎫	
Scissors or nail file	25	36 ⎭	+9·0

TABLE 6.4. *Time budget of daily activities, 1960 and 1964*

(Three hospitals; N = 233)

	Mean hours occupied per day	
Activity	1960	1964
In bed	10·9	10·6
Meals and toilet	2·7	2·5
Work and O.T.	4·1	4·6
Television and radio	1·0	1·2
Other leisure activities	1·0	1·6
Nothing	4·5	3·5
Total	24·2	24·0

TABLE 6.5. *Change in clinical categorisation, 1960–1964*
(Three hospitals; N = 233)

Clinical category in 1960	Category in 1964					Total
	1	2	3	4	5	
1 Moderate symptoms only	73	1	—	2	—	76
2 Coherent delusions predominant	14	8	1	—	—	23
3 Incoherence of speech predominant	9	5	22	2	3	41
4 Poverty of speech predominant	23	2	4	28	1	58
5 Mute or almost mute	3	1	5	5	21	35
Total	122	17	32	37	25	233

TABLE 6.6. *Ratings of four clinical symptoms in 1960 and 1964*
(Three hospitals; N = 233)

Symptom		Symptom rating		
		Minimal or none (1, 2) %	Moderate (3) %	Severe (4, 5) %
Flatness of affect	1960	11	21	68
	1964	20	30	50
Poverty of speech	1960	33	21	46
	1964	52	18	30
Incoherence of speech	1960	72	10	18
	1964	77	8	15
Coherently-expressed delusions	1960	77	5	18
	1964	71	18	11

TABLE 6.7. *Mean S.W. scores in 1960 and 1964*
within three improvement categories

(Three hospitals; N = 233)

			Mean S.W. score		Level of significance
	Clinical improvement category	N	1960	1964	
M	Group 1 in 1960 and 1964	73	2·0	1·7	N.S.
I	Groups 2–5 in 1960; improved in 1964	71	5·2	3·2	p < 0·001
NC	Groups 2–5 in 1960; no change or worse in 1964	89	6·3	5·5	N.S.

TABLE 6.8. *Relation between change in clinical category*
and change in S.W. score, 1960–1964

(Three hospitals; N = 233)

		Change in S.W. score			
		D 0–3 in 1960 and 1964	E 4+ in 1960, 0–3 in 1964	F 4+ in 1964	Total
Clinical improvement category					
M	Group 1 in 1960 and 1964	58	9	6	73
I	Groups 2–5 in 1960; improved in 1964	27	27	17	71
NC	Groups 2–5 in 1960; no change or worse in 1964	25	24	40	89
	Total	110	60	63	233

χ^2 (omitting groups M and D) = 5·92, df = 1, p < 0·05.

TABLE 6.9. *Ward behaviour in 1960 and 1964*

(Three hospitals; N = 233)

	1960			1964		
	0 %	1 %	2* %	0 %	1 %	2* %
Social withdrawal						
Slowness	65	20	15	72	18	10
Under-activity	63	21	16	76	17	7
Lack of conversation	46	43	11	46	46	8
Social withdrawal	37	33	30	40	40	20
Lack of leisure activity	41	40	19	49	38	13
Poor personal hygiene	64	25	11	73	22	5
Poor personal appearance	56	32	12	63	29	8
Poor meal-time behaviour	81	15	4	87	12	1
Socially embarrassing behaviour						
Over-activity	84	10	6	83	13	4
Laughing and talking to self	54	27	19	60	29	11
Posturing and mannerisms	71	15	14	80	11	9
Violence or threats	70	23	7	80	16	4

* The definitions of each rating are given in Appendix 2.2.

TABLE 6.10. *Clinical improvement 1960–1964 and length of stay*

(Three hospitals; N = 233)

Clinical improvement category	Length of stay (years)			Total
	2–10	11–20	21 +	
M Group 1 in 1960 and 1964	29	28	16	73
I Groups 2–5 in 1960; improved in 1964	26	28	17	71
NC Groups 2–5 in 1964; no change or worse in 1964	20	32	37	89
Total	75	88	70	233

χ^2 (I and NC) = 6·57, df = 2, p < 0·05.

TABLE 6.11. *Relation between social and clinical improvement, 1960–1964*

(Mean scores on five measures of social environment, 1960, and mean change in score between 1960 and 1964. Three hospitals; N = 233)

		Clinical improvement category		
Social variable	Maximum score possible	M Group 1 in 1960 and 1964 (N = 73)	I Groups 2–5 in 1960; improved in 1964 (N = 71)	NC Groups 2–5 in 1960; no change or worse in 1964 (N = 89)
Outside contact	15	7·5 +1·0*	4·8 +1·4**	4·0 +0·2
Favourable nurses' attitudes	13	9·4 +1·3*	6·5 +2·3***	4·9 +1·5***
Personal possessions	70	32·2 +3·2*	17·9 +11·0***	15·6 +5·8***
Occupation	15	6·0 +0·9*	4·0 +2·2***	4·2 +0·5
Time doing nothing (hours)	—	2·2 −0·1	5·7 −2·7***	5·4 −0·5

The significance of the change in score (based on 2×3 analyses of variance and subsequent t-tests) is indicated as follows:

* $p < 0.05$. ** $p < 0.01$. *** $p < 0.001$.

TABLE 6.12. *Decrease in time doing nothing, and change in clinical categorisation, 1960–1964*

(Three hospitals; N = 233)

Change in time doing nothing	Clinical improvement category			Total
	M	I	NC	
Group X: No change from low score	38	13	14	65
Group Y: Improved from high score	16	42	26	84
Group Z: No change from high score	19	16	49	84
Total	73	71	89	233

Omitting groups M and X; $\chi^2 = 18.5$, df = 1, p = < 0.001.

TABLE 6.13. *Decrease in time doing nothing, and change in S.W. score, 1960–1964*

(Three hospitals; N = 233)

Change in time doing nothing	Change in S.W. score			
	D 0–3 in 1960 and 1964	E 4+ in 1960, 0–3 in 1964	F 4+ in in 1964	Total
Group X: No change from low score	46	10	9	65
Group Y: Improved, from high score	32	30	22	84
Group Z: No change from high score	32	20	32	84
Total	110	60	63	233

Omitting groups D and X; $\chi^2 = 3 \cdot 85$, df = 1, p = < 0·05.

TABLE 6.14. *Change in time spent in various daily activities (hours), by patients in three clinical improvement groups*

(Three hospitals; N = 233)

Activity	Clinical improvement group			Mean change per individual
	M (N 73)	I (N 71)	NC (N 89)	
In bed	−0·44	−0·27	−0·13	−0·25
Meals and toilet	−0·13	−0·17	−0·18	−0·15
Work and O.T.	−0·41	+1·79	+0·24	+0·54
Television and radio	−0·12	+0·44	+0·21	+0·19
Other leisure activities	+0·93	+0·75	+0·32	+0·58
Time doing nothing	−0·09	−2·69	−0·51	−1·04

TABLE 6.15. *Change in attitude to discharge, 1960–1964*

(Three hospitals; N = 233)

	Attitude to discharge, 1964					
Attitude to discharge, 1960	1, 2	3	4	5	6, 7	Total
1, 2 Definite desire to leave	17	9	1	3	1	31
3 Ambivalent or vague	5	20	4	16	1	46
4 Indifferent	4	10	4	5	4	27
5 Desire to stay	1	12	1	53	4	71
6, 7 Not rated because in- coherent or mute	5	4	7	11	31	58
Total	32	55	17	88	41	233

TABLE 6.16. *Attitude to discharge and length of stay in 1960 and 1964*

(Three hospitals; N = 233)

		Length of stay in 1960 (years)			
Favourable attitudes (1–3)		2–10	11–20	21+	Total
1960	N	60	68	47	175
	% favourable	67	41	19	
1964	N	65	74	53	192
	% favourable	62	42	30	

Table 7.1   225

TABLE 7.1. *Change in 'poverty of the social environment' as measured by the mean scores on five variables in 1960 and 1964*

(Three hospitals separately; N = 233)

| | Maximum score possible | Mean scores in 1960 and 1964 | | | | | |
| | | Netherne (N = 85) | | Mapperley (N = 66) | | Severalls (N = 82) | |
		1960	1964	1960	1964	1960	1964
Outside contact	15	6·9	7·9**	6·4	6·3	2·9	4·2***
Favourable nurses' attitudes	13	9·1	9·7	6·6	8·0**	4·5	7·5***
Personal posses-sions	70	28·0	39·2***	27·1	21·4†††	10·2	21·8***
Occupation	15	6·0	6·8*	5·5	5·5	2·6	5·1***
Hours doing	—	3·4	3·0	3·4	3·5	6·5	3·9***

The significance of the change in score (based on 2×3 analyses of variance and subsequent t-tests) is indicated as follows:

Improvement: *⎫
Deterioration: †⎭ $p < 0.05$ **⎫ ††⎭ $p < 0.01$ ***⎫ †††⎭ $p < 0.01$.

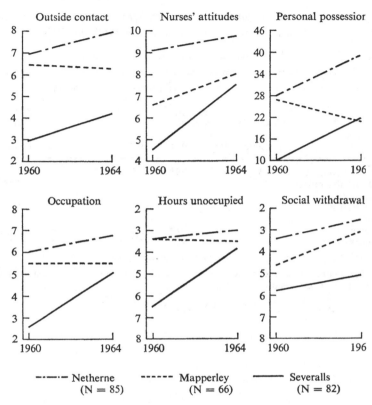

Fig. 7.2. Social and clinical change, 1960–1964.
(Three hospitals separately; N = 233.)

TABLE 7.3. *Changes in nurses' attitudes, 1960–1964*

(Three hospitals separately; N = 233)

	Netherne		Mapperley		Severalls	
	\% of patients					
	1960	1964	1960	1964	1960	1964
Could be on an open ward	93	100	100	98	91	100
Need not be certified	93	100	95	94	79	100*
Could have own clothes	89	99	90	85	48	74*
Knows the value of money	81	89	61	76*	33	57*
Could look after money	77	87	53	58	34	62*
Could do useful work in hospital	73	67	51	58	12	44**
Could go out to local shop	71	86*	47	62*	24	49*
Could have scissors	85	88	58	71*	45	67*
Could bath alone	72	78	41	76**	34	66**
Could have matches	76	81	26	51*	18	55**
Could go out with men	69	74	17	48**	18	50**
Could work outside hospital now	18	19	12	12	4	16
Could be discharged now	13	7	9	4	1	12
	(N = 85)		(N = 66)		(N = 82)	

* Increase of 15–29\%.   ** Increase of 30\% or more.

TABLE 7.4. *Changes in ownership of personal possessions, 1960–1964*

(Three hospitals separately; N = 233)

	Netherne		Mapperley		Severalls	
	\% of patients owning specified article(s)					
	1960	1964	1960	1964	1960	1964
Dress or suit	95	100	100	95	45	99***
Overcoat or raincoat	78	94*	97	92	23	98***
Brush, comb, etc.	87	100	68	97*	41	96***
Purse or handbag	76	93*	65	86*	37	61*
Toothbrush	86	96	59	76*	24	44*
Make-up materials	70	92*	54	38†	29	65**
Personal ornament	62	86*	62	58	24	52*
Mirror	49	65*	35	15†	5	24*
Scissors or nail file	50	69*	17	8	6	25*
	(N = 85)		(N = 66)		(N = 82)	

* Increase of 15–29\%.   ** Increase of 30–44\%.
*** Increase of 45\% or more.   † Decrease of 15\% or more.

TABLE 7.5. *Time budget of daily activities in 1960 and 1964*

(Three hospitals separately; N = 233)

| | Mean hours occupied per day | | | | | |
| | Netherne | | Mapperley | | Severalls | |
Activity	1960	1964	1960	1964	1960	1964
In bed	10·4	10·5	11·2	10·7	11·0	10·6
Meals and toilet	2·6	2·4	2·8	2·5	2·7	2·7
Work and O.T.	5·0	4·9	4·7	4·5	2·6	4·4
Television and radio	1·0	1·1	0·9	1·2	1·1	1·3
Other leisure activities	1·7	2·1	1·0	1·6	0·3	1·0
Nothing	3·4	3·0	3·4	3·5	6·5	3·9
Total	24·1	24·0	24·0	24·0	24·2	23·9
	(N = 85)		(N = 66)		(N = 82)	

TABLE 7.6. *Percentage of patients in various types of occupation in 1960 and 1964*

(Three hospitals separately; N = 233)

| | Netherne | | Mapperley | | Severalls | |
| | 1960 | 1964 | 1960 | 1964 | 1960 | 1964 |
Activity	%	%	%	%	%	%
Working outside hospital	2	8	7	6	0	1
Industrial work in hospital	26	31	2	0	0	13
Occupational therapy	4	8	14	38	26	32
Work in hospital department or another ward	39	22	37	17	14	12
Ward work	17	18	21	21	17	20
Virtually eunemployed*	12	13	19	19	43	22
	100	100	100	101	100	100
N =	100	85	73	66	100	82

* Total of 1½ hours or less occupied.

(N.B. If more than one activity, the chief one has been taken.)

TABLE 7.7. *Percentage of patients confined to ward,*
or visiting home, in 1960 and 1964

(Three hospitals separately; N = 233)

	Netherne		Mapperley		Severalls	
	1960	1964	1960	1964	1960	1964
Visits home occasionally	29	40	32	32	7	10
Confined to ward on day of survey	17	14	16	12	68	22
N =	100	85	73	66	100	82

TABLE 7.8. *Changes in ward restrictiveness score, 1960–1964*

(Three hospitals separately; N = 135)

(a) Netherne

Score in 1960	Score in 1964			Total
	0–9	10–29	30+	
0–9	25	3	0	28
10–29	11	4	1	16
30+	3	2	2	7
Total	39	9	3	51

(b) Mapperley

	0–9	10–29	30+	Total
0–9	4	0	0	4
10–29	15	24	0	39
30+	0	0	0	0
Total	19	24	0	43

(c) Severalls

	0–9	10–29	30+	Total
0–9	0	1	1	2
10–29	0	2	4	6
30+	0	14	19	33
Total	0	17	24	41

TABLE 7.9. *Number of patients in clinical categories, 1960–1964*
(Three hospitals separately; N = 233)

Clinical category in 1960	Clinical category in 1964					
	1	2	3	4	5	Total
(a) *Netherne*						
1 Moderate symptoms only	28	1	—	1	—	30
2 Coherent delusions predominant	9	4	1	—	—	14
3 Incoherence of speech predominant	2	—	11	1	3	17
4 Poverty of speech predominant	7	2	1	8	—	18
5 Mute or almost mute	—	—	2	1	3	6
Total	46	7	15	11	6	85
(b) *Mapperley*						
1 Moderate symptoms only	24	—	—	1	—	25
2 Coherent delusions predominant	4	2	—	—	—	6
3 Incoherence of speech predominant	1	3	5	1	—	10
4 Poverty of speech predominant	4	—	2	10	—	16
5 Mute or almost mute	—	—	1	1	7	9
Total	33	5	8	13	7	66
(c) *Severalls*						
1 Moderate symptoms only	21	—	—	—	—	21
2 Coherent delusions predominant	1	2	—	—	—	3
3 Incoherence of speech predominant	6	2	6	—	—	14
4 Poverty of speech predominant	12	—	1	10	1	24
5 Mute or almost mute	3	1	2	3	11	20
Total	43	5	9	13	12	82

TABLE 7.10. *Percentage of patients in clinical categories,*
1960–1964

(Three hospitals separately; N = 233)

	Clinical category	Netherne 1960 %	Netherne 1964 %	Mapperley 1960 %	Mapperley 1964 %	Severalls 1960 %	Severalls 1964 %
1a and 1b	Moderate symptoms only	26	51	32	47	22	38
1c	Moderate speech symptoms but severe flatness of affect	9	4	6	3	4	15
2	Coherent delusions predominant	17	8	9	8	4	6
3	Incoherence of speech predominant	20	18	15	12	17	11
4	Poverty of speech predominant	21	13	24	20	29	16
5	Mute or almost mute	7	7	14	11	24	15
	Total per cent	100	101	100	101	100	101
		(N = 85)		(N = 66)		(N = 82)	

TABLE 7.11. *Mean S.W. scores in 1960 and 1964, by*
'clinical improvement category'

(Three hospitals separately, N = 233)

		Mean S.W. scores					
		Netherne		Mapperley		Severalls	
	Clinical improvement category	1960	1964	1960	1964	1960	1964
M	Group 1 in 1960 and 1964	2·1 (N = 28)	1·1	2·1 (N = 24)	1·2	1·7 (N = 21)	3·0
I	Groups 2–5 in 1960; improved in 1964	2·8 (N = 24)	1·6	5·3 (N = 16)	2·9	7·0 (N = 31)	4·7
NC	Groups 2–5 in 1960; no change or worse in 1964	4·9 (N = 33)	4·4	6·7 (N = 26)	5·0	7·5 (N = 30)	7·1
	Total	3·4 (N = 85)	2·5	4·7 (N = 66)	3·1	5·8 (N = 82)	5·1

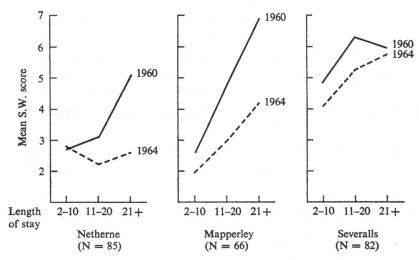

Fig. 7.12. Mean S.W. score in 1960 and 1964, by length of stay.
(Three hospitals separately; N = 233.)

Table 7.13   233

TABLE 7.13. *Individual items making up S.W. score in 1960 and 1964; percentages in each rating category*

(Three hospitals separately; N = 233)

		Netherne (N = 85)			Mapperley (N = 66)			Severalls (N = 82)		
		0 %	1 %	2* %	0 %	1 %	2* %	0 %	1 %	2* %
Slowness	1960	77	13	10	55	27	18	60	21	20
	1964	77	14	9	77	15	8	63	23	13
Under-activity	1960	76	15	9	56	36	8	56	15	29
	1964	77	17	6	82	15	3	70	18	12
Lack of con-	1960	51	45	3	53	35	12	34	48	18
versation	1964	58	40	2	55	39	6	26	60	15
Social withdrawal	1960	44	31	24	44	36	20	24	33	43
	1964	59	29	12	44	39	17	16	52	32
Lack of leisure	1960	48	33	20	41	44	15	33	45	22
interests	1964	64	27	9	59	26	15	26	60	15
Poor personal	1960	91	2	7	67	21	12	61	24	15
hygiene	1964	92	6	2	86	11	3	71	18	11
Poor personal	1960	76	21	3	46	44	11	43	35	22
appearance	1964	76	22	2	55	42	3	54	31	16
Poor meal-time	1960	92	7	1	71	29	2	79	16	5
behaviour	1964	93	6	1	86	14	0	81	17	2

* 0 = No abnormal behaviour   1 = Moderately abnormal   2 = Severely abnormal.

(See Appendix 2.2 for full details of scales.)

TABLE 7.14. *Individual items making up S.E. score in 1960 and 1964;*
percentages in each rating category

(Three hospitals separately; N = 233)

		Netherne (N = 85)			Mapperley (N = 66)			Severalls (N = 82)		
		0 %	1 %	2* %	0 %	1 %	2* %	0 %	1 %	2* %
Over-activity	1960	86	10	3	73	12	15	90	9	1
	1964	79	16	5	86	9	5	83	12	5
Lauging and	1960	66	19	15	38	36	26	55	28	17
talking to self	1964	67	27	6	59	30	11	54	29	17
Posturing and	1960	77	15	8	62	15	23	73	13	13
mannerisms	1964	83	7	10	80	11	9	77	15	9
Threats or	1960	78	20	2	56	35	9	73	17	10
violence	1964	79	20	1	73	24	3	87	9	5

* 0 = No abnormal behaviour   1 = Moderately abnormal   2 = Severely
abnormal.

(See Appendix 2.2 for full details of scales.)

TABLE 7.15. *Change in amount of time spent doing nothing,*
in three clinical improvement groups, 1960–1964

(Three hospitals separately; N = 233)

	Change in hours doing nothing		
Clinical improvement category	Netherne	Mapperley	Severalls
M Group 1 in 1960 and 1964	−0·2	+0·8	−0·8
I Groups 2–5 in 1960; improved in 1964	−1·0	−1·7*	−4·5***
NC Groups 2–5 in 1960; no change or worse in 1964	−0·1	+0·5	−1·8**

The significance of the change in score (based on 3 separate 2×3 analyses of
variance, and subsequent t-tests) is indicated as follows:

Improvement: *$\}$ $p < 0.05$ **$\}$ $p < 0.01$ ***$\}$ $p < 0.001$
Deterioration: †$\}$ ††$\}$ †††$\}$

The change in group I at Netherne is significant at the 10 % level.

TABLE 7.16. *Outcome in January 1968: by hospital*

(N = 273)

Outcome	Netherne N	Mapperley N	Mapperley %	Severalls N	Total N	Total %
Dead	7	10	13·7	8	25	9·2
In-patient	64	47	64·4	64	175	64·1
Transferred to another hospital	2	—	—	2	4	1·5
Living in hospital, but working out	8	—	—	—	8	2·9
Attending as day patient	—	8*	11·0	—	8	2·9
Discharged and still out**	19	8	11·0	26	53	19·4
Total	100	73	100·1	100	273	100·0

* Living in hospital-supervised hostels.
** Including patients in hostels, part III accommodation, boarding out and in living-in domestic work.

TABLE 7.17. *Characteristics differentiating fifty-three patients, discharged and not in hospital in January 1968, from the remaining group*

(Three hospitals; N = 273)

Characteristic	Discharged patients %	Remaining patients %
Father's occupation: non-manual	43·4	33·7
Marital status: ever-married	30·2	25·0
Length of stay (1960): under 10 years	45·3	31·8
Clinical classification (1960): groups 1–3	62·2	29·2
Social withdrawal (1960): score 0–3	83·1	43·6
General knowledge (1960): full score	62·3	29·6
Attitude to discharge (1960): some desire to leave	58·5	33·2
Favourable nurses' attitudes (1960): score 11 +	54·7	24·1
Contact with outside (1960): score 8 +	41·5	25·5
	(N = 53)	(N = 220)

TABLE 7.18. *Relationship between clinical improvement in severely impaired patients and subsequent discharge*

(Three hospitals; groups I and NC only; N = 160)

		Whether discharged after 1964 or not		
	Clinical improvement category	Discharged	Not discharged	Total
I	Groups 2–5 in 1960; improved in 1964	12	59	71
NC	Groups 2–5 in 1960; no change or worse in 1964	2	87	89
	Total	14	146	160

$\chi^2 = 10.67$, df = 1, p < 0.001.

TABLE 7.19. *Patients rated in 1968, by age in 1960*

(Three hospitals separately; N = 191)

Age in 1960	Netherne		Mapperley		Severalls		Total
	N	%	N	%	N	%	
–39	14	19·4	9	16·4	18	28·1	41
40–49	27	37·5	15	27·3	18	28·1	60
50–59	31	43·1	31	56·4	28	43·8	90
Total	72	100·0	55	100·1	64	100·0	191

Table 7.20–Figure 7.21 237

TABLE 7.20. *Patients rated in 1968, by length of stay in 1960*
(Three hospitals separately; N = 191)

Length of stay in 1960 (years)	Netherne		Mapperley		Severalls		Total
	N	%	N	%	N	%	
2–5	12	16·7	5	9·1	7	10·9	24
6–10	16	22·2	11	20·0	12	18·8	39
11–20	25	34·7	18	32·7	24	37·5	67
21+	19	26·4	21	38·2	21	32·8	61
Total	72	100·0	55	100·0	64	100·0	191

χ^2 (combining groups 2–10) = 4·00, df = 4, p = > 0·05.

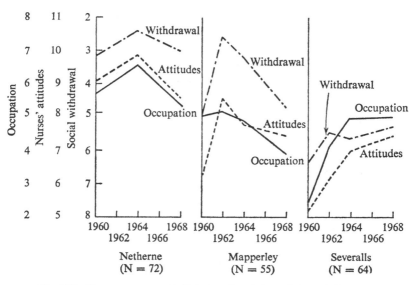

Fig. 7.21. Three measures of clinical and social condition, 1960–1968.
(Three hospitals separately; N = 191.)

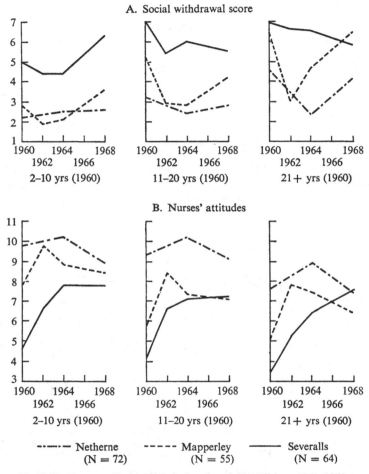

Fig. 7.22. Four measures of clinical and social condition, 1960–1968, by length of stay in 1960. (Three hospitals separately; N = 191.)

Figure 7.22 239

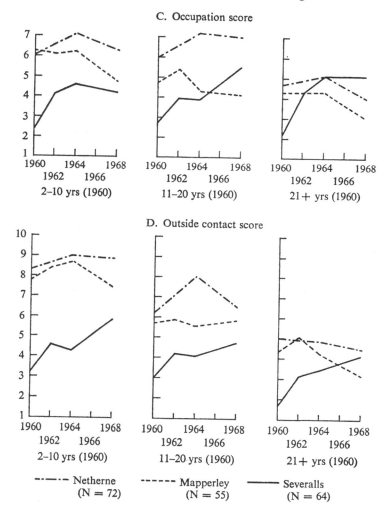

C. Occupation score

2–10 yrs (1960)   11–20 yrs (1960)   21+ yrs (1960)

D. Outside contact score

2–10 yrs (1960)   11–20 yrs (1960)   21+ yrs (1960)

—·—·— Netherne   -------- Mapperley   ——— Severalls
(N = 72)   (N = 55)   (N = 64)

TABLE 7.23. *Relationship between change in S.W. score**
and change in occupation score

(Mapperley Hospital 1962–1968; N = 5)

Change in S.W. score*	Change in occupation score					
	+2 or more	+1	0	−1	−2 or more	Total
+2 or more	1	—	1	1	2	5
+1	1	1	—	—	1	3
0	2	—	4	1	4	11
−1	3	—	—	2	2	7
−2 or more	3	1	3	2	20	29
Total	10	2	8	6	29	55

When each variable is split close to the median (between −1 and −2), $\chi^2 = 6.98$, df = 1, p < 0.01.

* The sign of the change in S.W. score has been reversed, so that ' + ' means an improvement in the case of each score, and ' − ' means a deterioration.

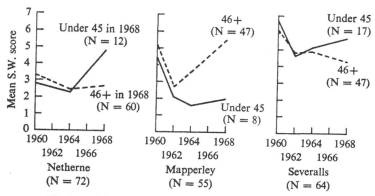

Fig. 7.24. Mean S.W. scores in two age groups, 1960–1968.
(Three hospitals separately; N = 191.)

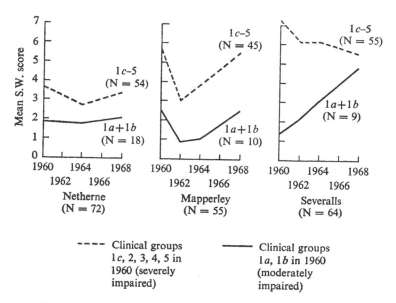

Fig. 7.25. Mean S.W. score, 1960–1968, by clinical groups, 1960.
(Three hospitals separately; N = 191.)

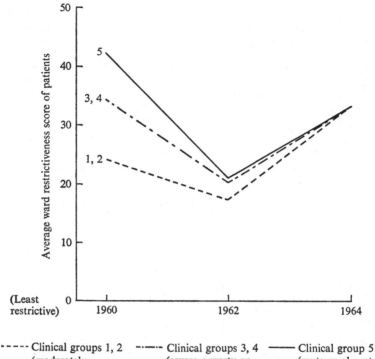

Fig. 7.26. Relationship of ward restrictiveness to mental state
at Severalls in 1960, 1962 and 1964.

Figure 7.27   243

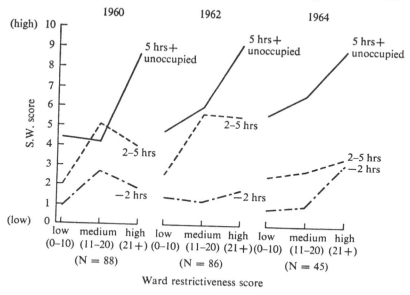

Fig. 7.27. Relationship of S.W. scores, time spent unoccupied and ward restrictiveness in 1960, 1962 and 1964. (Three hospitals; N = 219.)

TABLE 7.28. *Clinical improvement at Severalls between 1960 and 1964 and changes in ward restrictiveness and amount of time spent unoccupied*

$(N = 39)$

| Change between 1960–1964 | | | | |
Time doing nothing reduced by at least 2 hours	Ward restrictiveness reduced by at least 20 %	Improved	Not improved	Proportion improved
(a) Mental state				
Yes	Yes	9	1	0·90
Yes	No	9	5	0·64
No	Yes	3	5	0·37
No	No	1	6	0·14
		$p < 0.05$, $\chi^2 = 11.43$, 3 df.		
(b) Social withdrawal				
Yes	Yes	7	3	0·70
Yes	No	5	9	0·36
No	Yes	2	6	0·25
No	No	0	7	0·00
		$p < 0.05$, $\chi^2 = 9.35$, 3 df.		

Note:
1. Social withdrawal improvement = 2 points or more.
2. All moderately-handicapped patients in 1960 excluded.

TABLE 7.29. *Changes in drug administration and clinical change, 1960–1964*

(Mapperley and Severalls hospitals; N = 158)

| | Clinical improvement category | | | | | |
| | M Group 1 in 1960 and 1962 | | I Groups 2–5 in 1960; improved in 1962 | | NC Groups 2–5 in 1960; no change or worse in 1962 | |
	Mapperley	Severalls	Mapperley	Severalls	Mapperley	Severalls
No drug throughout	2	3	2	5	4	3
Stopped drug treatment	0	0	0	2	0	3
Same drug throughout	12	4	4	7	7	11
Minor change in dose or type of drug	8	4	4	2	6	5
Major change in dose or type of drug	3	8	4	6	7	6
Began drug treatment	1	0	1	9	2	12
Total	26	19	15	31	26	40

TABLE 9.1. *Length of stay of patients in Columbia County and Mapperley hospitals*

Length of stay (years)	Columbia County 1964 %	Mapperley 1960 %
2–10	46	29
11–20	43	34
21+	11	37
	N = 38	N = 73

TABLE 9.2. *Clinical classification of patients in Columbia County and Mapperley hospitals, 1964*

	Clinical category	Columbia County Hospital			Mapperley Women %
		Men N	Women N	Total %	
1a	No florid symptoms, poverty of speech or flatness of affect	2	3	13	27
1b	Moderate symptoms only	5	5	26	20
1c	Moderate speech symptoms but severe flatness of affect	4	—	11	3
2	Coherent delusions predominant	2	4	16	8
3	Incoherence of speech predominant	2	4	16	12
4	Poverty of speech predominant	2	3	13	20
5	Mute or almost mute	—	2	5	11
	Total N	17	21	38	66

TABLE 9.3. *Attitude to discharge of patients in Columbia County and Mapperley hospitals, 1964*

	Columbia County Hospital			Mapperley Women %
	Men N	Women N	Total %	
Definite wish to leave	—	5	13	12
Definite wish to leave but qualified	2	1	8	3
Ambivalent or vague	5	4	24	23
Indifferent	2	6	21	21
Wish to stay	8	5	34	41
Total N	17	21	38	66

TABLE 9.4. *Personal possessions of patients in Columbia County and Mapperley hospitals, 1964*

	Columbia County Hospital			Mapperley Women %
	Men N	Women N	Total %	
Dress, suit, etc.	16	21	97	95
Overcoat etc.	15	15	79	92
Comb or hairbrush	14	17	82	97
Make-up	—	14	67	38
Toothbrush	7	18	66	76
Scissors or nail file	15	10	66	8
Mirror	—	11	52	15
Purse or handbag	—	13	62	86
Personal ornament	—	13	62	58
Total N	17	21	38	66

TABLE 9.5. *Attitudes of nurses at Columbia County and Mapperley hospitals, 1964*

	Columbia County Hospital			Mapperley Women %
	Men N	Women N	Total %	
Could do useful work in hospital	15	17	84	58
Could work outside while living in	5	7	32	12
Could be discharged now	1	4	13	4
Could appreciate the value of money	11	5	42	76
Could be trusted with matches	15	5	53	51
Could be trusted with scissors	14	12	68	71
Could be on an open ward	15	14	76	98
Could bath without supervision	15	17	84	76
Need not be committed	—	—	—	94
Could go out with patient of opposite sex	15	5 (24%)	53	48
Could go to local shop	12	8	53	62
Total N	17	21	38	66

TABLE 9.6. *Contact with the outside, at Columbia County and Mapperley hospitals, 1964*

| During past six months | Columbia County Hospital | | | Mapperley Women % |
	Men N	Women N	Total %	
Visited:				
Once a month or more	3	3	16	20
Less than once a month	7	8	39	23
Never	7	10	45	58
Goes home:				
Once a month or more	1	2	8	23
Less than once a month	4	1	13	8
Never	12	18	79	70
Parole:				
Restricted to ward unless escorted	2	18 ⎫ (95%)	53	12
Allowed out in supervised working party	0	2 ⎭	5	0
Ground privileges	15	1 (5%)	42	53
Town privileges	0	0	0	35
Total N	17	21	38	66
Summary score	5·06	1·95	3·41	6·26

TABLE 9.7. *Average time budget (hours) at Columbia County and Mapperley hospitals, 1964*

| | Columbia County Hospital | | | Mapperley |
	Men	Women	Total	
In bed	9·0	9·8	9·4	10·7
Toilet and meals	2·3	2·5	2·4	2·5
Employment:				
Ward work	0·5	1·2	0·9	1·5
Occupational therapy	0·2	0·4	0·3	1·7
Work off ward	5·8	2·2	3·8	1·3
Leisure:				
TV and radio	1·8	2·2	2·1	1·2
Other	1·2	1·3	1·3	1·6
Nothing	3·3	4·3	3·8	3·5
Total hours	24·1	23·9	24·0	24·0
Total N	17	21	38	66

Table 9.8　249

TABLE 9.8. *Clinical classification of thirty-eight patients in Columbia County and Mapperley hospitals, matched for length of stay, 1964*

	Clinical category	Columbia County Hospital		Mapperley	
		N	%	N	%
1a	No florid symptoms, poverty of speech or flatness of affect	5	13	13	34
1b	Moderate symptoms only	10	26	9	24
1c	Moderate speech symptoms but severe flatness of affect	4	11	2	5
2	Coherent delusions predominant	6	16	3	8
3	Incoherence of speech predominant	6	16	6	16
4	Poverty of speech predominant	5	13	3	8
5	Mute or almost mute	2	5	2	5
	Total	38	100	38	100

REFERENCES

Achté, K. A. (1961). The course of schizophrenic and schizophreniform psychoses. *Acta psychiatrica et neurologica Scandinavica.* Supplement 155, 273.

Barton, R. (1959). *Institutional Neurosis.* Bristol: Wright.

Barton, R. (1966). Developing a service for elderly demented patients,Chap. 26, *Psychiatric Hospital Care.* London: Bailliere, Tindall and Cassell.

Belknap, I. (1956). *Human Problems of a State Mental Hospital.* New York: McGraw Hill.

Bell, G. M. (1955). A mental hospital with open doors. *Int. J. soc. Psychiat.* 1, 42.

Bennett, D. H. and Wing, J. K. (1963). Sheltered workshops for the psychiatrically handicapped. In: *Trends in the Mental Health Services.* (Eds.) H. Freeman and J. Farndale. Oxford: Pergamon Press.

Bennett, D. H., Folkard, S. and Nicholson, A. K. (1961). Resettlement Unit in a mental hospital. *Lancet* 2, 539.

Birley, J. L. T. and Brown, G. W. (1970). Crises and life changes preceding the onset or relapse of acute schizophrenia: clinical aspects. *Brit. J. Psychiat.* 116, 327.

Bockoven, J. S. (1956). Moral treatment in American psychiatry. *J. nerv. ment. Dis.* 124, 167.

Brooke, Eileen (1957). A national study of schizophrenic patients in relation to occupation. *Int. Congr. Psychiat.* 3, 52.

Brown, G. W. (1960a). Length of hospital stay and schizophrenia: a review of statistical studies. *Acta psychiat. neurol. scand.* 35, 414.

Brown, G. W. (1960b). Social factors influencing length of hospital stay of schizophrenic patients. *Brit. med. J.* 2, 1300.

Brown, G. W. and Birley, J. L. T. (1968). Crises and life changes and the onset of schizophrenia. *J. of Health and Soc. Behavior* 9, 203.

Brown, G. W. and Wing, J. K. (1962). A comparative clinical and social survey of three mental hospitals. *Sociological Studies in the British National Health Service* (Sociological Review Monograph No. 5, ed. P. Halmos). University of Keele.

Brown, G. W., Bone, M., Dalison, B. and Wing, J. K. (1966). *Schizophrenia and Social Care: A Comparative Follow-up of 339 Schizophrenic Patients.* Maudsley Monograph No. 17. London: Oxford University Press.

Brown, G. W., Monck, E., Carstairs, G. M. and Wing, J. K. (1962). The influence of family life on the course of schizophrenic illness. *Brit. J. prev. soc. med.* 16, 55.

Calwell, W. P. K., Jacobsen, M. and Skarbek, A. (1964). A comparative study of oxypertine and trifluoperazine in chronic schizophrenia. *Brit. J. Psychiat.* 110, 520.

Carse, J., Panton, N. E. and Watt, A. (1958). The Worthing experiment. *Lancet* 1, 39.

Carstairs, G. M., O'Connor, N. and Rawnsley, K. (1956). The organization of a hospital workshop for chronic psychotic patients. *Brit. J. prev. soc. Med.* 10, 136.

Cartwright, Ann (1964). *Human Relations and Hospital Care.* London: Routledge & Kegan Paul.

Catterson, A., Bennett, D. H. and Freudenberg, R. K. (1963). A survey of longstay schizophrenic patients. *Brit. J. Psychiat.* 109, 750.

Clark, D. H. (1956). Functions of the mental hospital. *Lancet* 2, 1005.

Clark, D. H. (1964). *Administrative Therapy.* London: Tavistock Publications.

Clark, D. H. (1965). The therapeutic community—concept, practice and future. *Brit. J. Psychiat.* 111, 947.

Clark, D. H., Hooper, D. F. and Oram, E. G. (1961). Creating a therapeutic community in a psychiatric ward. *Human Relations* 15, 123.

Collins, A. D. and Dundas, J. (1967). A double-blind trial of amitriptyline-perphenazine, perphenazine and placebo in chronic withdrawn inert schizophrenics. *Brit. J. Psychiat.* 113, 1425.

Conolly, J. (1856). *The Treatment of the Insane without Mechanical Restraints.* London: Smith, Elder & Co.

Cooper, B. (1961). Social class and prognosis in schizophrenia. *Brit. J. prev. soc. Med.* 15, 17.

Deutsch, A. (1949). *The Mentally Ill in America.* New York: Columbia University Press.

Dunham, H. W. (1965). *Community and Schizophrenia.* Detroit: Wayne State University Press.

Dunham, H. W. and Weinburg, S. K. (1960). *Culture of the State Mental Hospital.* Detroit: Wayne State University Press.

Early, D. F. (1960). The Industrial Therapy Organisation (Bristol): a development of work in hospital. *Lancet* 2, 754.

Early, D. F. (1965). Domestic and Economic Rehabilitation. In: *Psychiatric Hospital Care.* London: Bailliere, Tindall & Cassell.

Ekdawi, M. Y. (1966). Changes in ward behaviour of severely disabled schizophrenic patients. *Brit. J. Psychiat.* 112, 265.

Ekdawi, M. Y., Rogers, W., Slaughter, R. S. and Bennett, D. H. (1968). A patients' record office in a mental hospital occupational programme. *Brit. J. Psychiat.* 114, 1305.

Ellenberger, H. F. (1960). Zoological garden and mental hospital. *Canad. Psychiat. Ass. J.* 5, 136.

Etzioni, A. (1961). *A Comparative Analysis of Complex Organisations.* New York: Free Press.

Festinger, L. (1957). *A Theory of Cognitive Dissonance.* Evanston: Row, Peterson.

Festinger, L. and Kelly, H. H. (1951). *Changing Attitudes Through Social Contacts.* Research Center for Group Dynamics, Institute for Social Research. University of Michigan.

Folkard, M. S. (1956). A sociological contribution to the understanding of aggression and its treatment. *Proc. Roy. Soc. Med.* **49**, 1030.

Foulds, G. A. and Dixon, Penelope (1962). The nature of intellectual deficit in schizophrenia. *Brit. J. soc. clin. Psychol.* **1**, 199.

Freeman, J., Mandelbrote, B. and Waldron, J. (1965). Attitudes to discharge among long-stay mental hospital patients and their relation to social and clinical factors. *Brit. J. soc. clin. Psychol.* **4**, 270.

Freeman, T., Cameron, J. L. and McGhie, A. (1958). *Chronic Schizophrenia*. London: Tavistock Publications.

Freudenberg, R. K. (1967). Theory and practice of the rehabilitation of the psychiatrically disabled. *Psychiat. Quart.* **41**, 698.

Freudenberg, R. K., Bennett, D. H. and May, A. R. (1957). The relative importance of physical and community methods in the treatment of schizophrenia. *Int. Congr. Psychiat.* **1**, 157.

Goffman, E. (1961). *Asylums: Essays on the Social Situation of Mental Patients and Other Inmates*. New York: Doubleday.

Goldberg, E. M. and Morrison, S. L. (1963). Schizophrenia and social class. *Brit. J. Psychiat.* **109**, 785.

Gottfries, I., Karlsson, K., Olsson, M. and Ramsing, H. (1968). Improvement of severely ill long-stay schizophrenic patients. *Social Psychiatry* **3**, 65.

Gruenberg, E. M. (Ed.) (1966). *Evaluating the Effectiveness of Community Mental Health Services*. New York: Milbank Mem. Fund.

Hall, J. and Moser, C. (1954). The social grading of occupations. In: *Social Mobility in Britain*. (Ed.) D. V. Glass. London: Routledge.

Hamilton, V. (1964). Psychological changes in chronic schizophrenics following differential activity programmes: a repeat study. *Brit. J. Psychiat.* **109**, 283.

Hamilton, V. and Salmon, P. (1962). Psychological changes in chronic schizophrenics following differential activity programmes. *J. ment. Sci.* **108**, 505.

Hare, E. H. (1956). Mental illness and social conditions in Bristol. *J. ment. Sci.* **102**, 349.

Hewitt, M. (1949). The unemployed disabled man. *Lancet* **2**, 523.

Hollingshead, A. B. and Redlich, F. C. (1958). *Social Class and Mental Illness*. New York: John Wiley & Sons.

Hooper, D. F. (1962). Changing the milieu in a psychiatric ward. *Human Relations* **15**, 111.

Hunt, P. V. (1967). A comparison of the effects of Oxypertine and Trifluoperazine in withdrawn schizophrenics. *Brit. J. Psychiat.* **113**, 1419.

Jones, K. (1954). *Lunacy Law and Conscience: 1744–1845*. London: Routledge.

Jones, K. (1960). *Mental Health and Social Policy: 1845–1959*. London: Routledge.

Jones, K. and Sidebotham, R. (1962). *Mental Hospitals at Work*. London: Routledge.

Jones, M. (1952). *Social Psychiatry: A Study of Therapeutic Communities.* London: Tavistock.

Jones, M. (1962). *Social Psychiatry in the Community, in Hospitals and in Prisons.* Springfield: Thomas.

Jones, M. (1966). Group work in mental hospitals. *Brit. J. Psychiat.* **112**, 1007.

Jones, M. (1968). *Beyond the Therapeutic Community.* New Haven: Yale University Press.

Kety, S. (1959). Biochemical theories of schizophrenia. *Science* **129**, 1528.

King, R. D. and Raynes, N. (1968*a*). An operational measure of inmate management in residential institutions. *Soc. Sci. and Med.* **2**, 41.

King, R. D. and Raynes, N. (1968*b*). Patterns of institutional care for the severely subnormal. *Amer. J. Ment. Def.* **72**, 700.

Kushlick, A. (1966). A community service for the mentally subnormal. *Soc. Psychiat.* **1**, 73.

Lemert, E. M. (1951). *Social Pathology.* New York: McGraw Hill.

Letemendia, F., Harris, A. D. and Willems, P. J. A. (1967). The clinical effects on a population of chronic schizophrenic patients of administrative changes in hospital. *Brit. J. Psychiat.* **113**, 959.

Macmillan, D. (1956). An integrated mental health service. *Lancet* **2**, 1094.

Macmillan, D. (1957). Hospital–Community Relationships. *Proceedings of the Thirty-Fourth Annual Conference of the Milbank Memorial Fund.* New York.

Macmillan, D. (1958*a*). Mental health services of Nottingham. *Int. J. Soc. Psychiat.* **4**, 5.

Macmillan, D. (1958*b*). Community treatment of mental illness. *Lancet* **2**, 201.

Macmillan, D. (1960). Preventive geriatrics. *Lancet* **2**, 1439.

Macmillan, D. (1961). Nuffield House: A Day Centre for the psychiatric elderly. *Gerontologia Clinica*, **3**, 133.

Macmillan, D. (1963). Recent developments in community mental health. *Lancet* **1**, 567.

Macmillan, D. (1967). Problems of a geriatric mental health service. *Brit. J. Psychiat.* **113**, 175.

Martin, D. V. (1962). *Adventure in Psychiatry.* London: Cassirer.

Mechanic, D. (1968). *Medical Sociology: A Selective View.* New York: Free Press.

Morgan, R. (1967). The personal orientation of long-stay psychiatric patients. *Brit. J. Psychiat.* **113**, 847.

Morgan, R. and Cushing, D. (1966). The personal possessions of long-stay patients in mental hospitals. *Soc. Psychiat.* **1**, 151.

Norris, Vera (1956). A statistical study of the influence of marriage on the hospital care of the mentally sick. *J. ment. Sci.* **102**, 467.

Ødegaard, Ø. (1946). Marriage and mental disease. *J. ment. Sci.* **92**, 35.

Ødegaard, Ø. (1953). New data on marriage and mental disease. *J. ment. Sci.* **99**, 778.

Olshansky, S., Grob, S. and Malamud, Irene (1958). Employers' attitudes and practices in the hiring of ex-mental patients. *Ment. Hyg.* **42**, 391.

Opler, M. (1967). *Culture and Social Psychiatry.* New York: Atherton Press.

Oram, E. G. and Knowles, M. C. (1964). The chronically mentally ill— movements in a rural area: 1900–1961. Chapter in *Problems and Progress in Medical Care.* (Ed.) G. McLachlan. London: Oxford University Press.

Philip, A. E. and McKechnie, A. A. (1969). The assessment of long-stay psychiatric patients. *Soc. Psychiat.* **4**, 66.

Piercy Report, see *Report of the Committee of Inquiry on the Rehabilitation, Training and Resettlement of Disabled Persons.*

Rapoport, R. N. (1960). *Community as Doctor.* London: Tavistock.

Rees, T. P. (1957). Back to moral treatment. *J. ment. Sci.* **103**, 303.

Report of the Committee of Inquiry on the Rehabilitation, Training and Resettlement of Disabled Persons (Piercy Report) (1956). Cmd. 9883. London: H.M.S.O.

Revans, R. W. (1962). Hospital Attitudes and Communication. In: *Sociological Review Monographs* No. 5. (Ed.) P. Halmos. University of Keele.

Rubenstein, R. and Lasswell, H. D. (1966). *The Sharing of Power in a Psychiatric Hospital.* New Haven: Yale University Press.

Scheff, T. (1963). The role of the mentally ill and the dynamics of mental disorder. *Sociometry,* **26**, 436.

Scheff, T. (1964). The societal reaction to deviance. *Social Problems,* **2**, 401.

Skarbek, A. and Hill, G. B. (1967). An extended trial of oxypertine in five selected cases of chronic schizophrenia. *Brit. J. Psychiat.* **113**, 1107.

Smith, K., Pumphrey, M. and Hall, J. O. (1963). The 'Last Straw': the decisive incidents resulting in the request for hospitalisation in 100 schizophrenic patients. *Amer. J. Psychiat.* **120**, 228.

Sommer, R. (1959). Patients who grow old in a mental hospital. *Geriatrics,* **14**, 581.

Stanton, A. and Schwartz, M. (1954). *The Mental Hospital.* New York: Basic Books.

Stone, A. A. and Eldred, S. H. (1959). Delusion formation during the activation of chronic schizophrenic patients. *Arch. gen. Psychiat.* **1**, 77.

Storey, P. B. (1966). Lumbar air encephalography in chronic schizophrenia: a controlled experiment. *Brit. J. Psychiat.* **112**, 135.

Titmuss, R. M. (1959). Community care as a challenge. *The Times,* 12 May 1959.

Tizard, J. (1964). *Community Services for the Mentally Handicapped.* London: Oxford University Press.

Tizard, J., King, R., Raynes, N. and Yule, W. (1966). The care and treatment of subnormal children in residential institutions. In: *What is Special Education?* Proceedings of the First International Conference of the Association for Special Education, July 1966. Pp. 164–176.

Townsend, P. (1962). *The Last Refuge.* London: Routledge.

Ullman, L. P. (1967). *Institution and Outcome*. London: Pergamon.

Venables, P. H. (1957). A short scale for 'activity-withdrawal' in schizophrenics. *J. ment. Sci.* **103**, 197.

Venables, P. H. (1960). The effect of auditory and visual stimulation on the skin potential response of schizophrenics. *Brain*, **83**, 77.

Venables, P. H. (1967). The relation of two-flash and two-click thresholds in schizophrenic and normal subjects. *Quart. J. exp. Psychol.* **18**, 371.

Venables, P. H. (1968). Experimental Psychological Studies of Chronic Schizophrenia. In: *Studies in Psychiatry*. (Eds.) M. Shepherd and D. L. Davies. London: Oxford University Press.

Venables, P. H. and O'Connor, N. (1959). A short scale of rating paranoid schizophrenia. *J. ment. Sci.* **105**, 815.

Venables, P. H. and Wing, J. K. (1962). Level of arousal and the subclassification of schizophrenics. *Arch. gen. Psychiat.* **7**, 114.

Wadsworth, W. V., Scott, R. F. and Tonge, W. L. (1958). A hospital workshop. *Lancet* **2**, 896.

Wardle, C. (1962). Social factors in the major functional psychoses. In: *Society: Problems and Methods of Study*. (Eds.) A. T. Welford, *et al.* London: Routledge.

Whitehead, J. A. (1965). A comprehensive psycho-geriatric service. *Lancet* **2**, 583.

Wing, J. K. (1960). A pilot experiment on the rehabilitation of long-hospitalised male schizophrenic patients. *Brit. J. prev. soc. Med.* **14**, 173.

Wing, J. K. (1961). A simple and reliable subclassification of chronic schizophrenia. *J. ment. Sci.* **107**, 862.

Wing, J. K. (1962). Institutionalism in mental hospitals. *Brit. J. soc. clin. Psychol.* **1**, 38.

Wing, J. K. (1963). Rehabilitation of psychiatric patients. *Brit. J. Psychiat.* **109**, 635.

Wing, J. K. (Ed.) (1966*a*). *Early Childhood Autism*. Oxford: Pergamon Press.

Wing, J. K. (1966*b*). Social and psychological changes in a rehabilitation unit. *Soc. Psychiat.* **1**, 21.

Wing, J. K. (1967). The concept of handicap in psychiatry. *Int. J. Psychiat.* **3**, 243.

Wing, J. K. and Brown, G. W. (1961). Social treatment of chronic schizophrenia: a comparative survey of three mental hospitals. *J. ment. Sci.* **107**, 847.

Wing, J. K. and Freudenberg, R. K. (1961). The response of severely ill chronic schizophrenic patients to social stimulation. *Amer. J. Psychiat.* **118**, 311.

Wing, J. K., Bennett, D. H. and Denham, J. (1964). *The Industrial Rehabilitation of Long-stay Schizophrenic patients*. Medical Research Council Memo. No. 42. London: H.M.S.O.

Wing, J. K., Monck, E., Brown, G. W. and Carstairs, G. M. (1964).

Morbidity in the community of schizophrenic patients discharged from London mental hospitals in 1959. *Brit. J. Psychiat.* **110**, 10.

Wing, J. K., Wing, L., and Hailey, A. (1970). The use of case registers for evaluating and planning psychiatric services. In: *Psychiatric Case Registers*. (Eds.) J. K. Wing, and R. Bransby. Dept. of Health Stat. Rep. Series. London: H.M.S.O.

Wing, L. (1956). The use of reserpine in chronic psychotic patients: a controlled trial. *J. ment. Sci.* **102**, 530.

Ytrehus, Å. (1959). Environmental therapy of chronic schizophrenic patients. *Acta Psychiat. Neurol.* **34**, 126.

Zusman, J. (1966). Some explanations of the changing appearance of psychotic patients. *Milbank Mem. Fund Quart.* **44**, 363.

SUBJECT INDEX

NAME INDEX